AF891288

An Atlas Illustrating
HIV in Dermatology

An Atlas Illustrating
HIV in Dermatology

Bela J Shah MD (Skin and VD)
Professor and Head
Department of Dermatology, STD and Leprosy
BJ Medical College
Ahmedabad, Gujarat, India

Foreword
FE Bilimoria

JAYPEE BROTHERS MEDICAL PUBLISHERS (P) LTD
New Delhi • London • Philadelphia • Panama

Jaypee Brothers Medical Publishers (P) Ltd.

Headquarters
Jaypee Brothers Medical Publishers (P) Ltd.
4838/24, Ansari Road, Daryaganj
New Delhi 110 002, India
Phone: +91-11-43574357
Fax: +91-11-43574314
Email: jaypee@jaypeebrothers.com

Overseas Offices

J.P. Medical Ltd.
83, Victoria Street, London
SW1H 0HW (UK)
Phone: +44-2031708910
Fax: +02-03-0086180
Email: info@jpmedpub.com

Jaypee-Highlights Medical Publishers Inc.
City of Knowledge, Bld. 237, Clayton
Panama City, Panama
Phone: +507-301-0496
Fax: +507-301-0499
Email: cservice@jphmedical.com

Jaypee Brothers Medical Publishers Ltd.
The Bourse
111 South Independence Mall East
Suite 835, Philadelphia, PA 19106, USA
Phone: + 267-519-9789
Email: joe.rusko@jaypeebrothers.com

Jaypee Brothers Medical Publishers (P) Ltd.
17/1-B, Babar Road, Block-B
Shaymali, Mohammadpur
Dhaka-1207, Bangladesh
Mobile: +08801912003485
Email: jaypeedhaka@gmail.com

Jaypee Brothers Medical Publishers (P) Ltd.
Shorakhute
Kathmandu, Nepal
Phone: +00977-9841528578
Email: jaypee.nepal@gmail.com

Website: www.jaypeebrothers.com
Website: www.jaypeedigital.com

Inquiries for bulk sales may be solicited at: jaypee@jaypeebrothers.com

An Atlas Illustrating HIV in Dermatology

First Edition: **2013**

ISBN 978-93-5025-050-1

Printed at: Ajanta Offset & Packagings Ltd., New Delhi

Dedicated to

My reward teacher and mentor
Dr Bharat H Shah

Foreword

According to the 2011-2012 estimate, India has 2 to 3 millions people living with HIV/AIDS. India's national epidemic is made up of a number of local epidemics, which vary even within the same state.

A clinician must be able to understand that sexually transmitted infection (STI) is a very important cofactor in HIV transmission as well as acquisition. STI management approaches are simplified by National AIDS Control Organization (NACO) training programs on enhanced syndromic management.

It is very important to understand the examination of the largest organ of the body, i.e. skin in relation to HIV. The HIV epidemic is mature enough now. The primary and secondary mucocutaneous manifestations seen in people living with HIV/AIDS (PLHA) provide an opportunity not only to identify the HIV, for the very first time, but also to classify them as per WHO staging and even institute ART.

Through this book, the author has aptly tried to present the clinical spectrum of HIV/AIDS. The varied collection of colored clinical photographs create a perfect image and understanding of the disease.

FE Bilimoria
Professor and Head
Department of Dermatology
SBKS Medical College
Vadodara, Gujarat, India

Preface

The first case of HIV in India was reported in the year 1986. As a postgraduate then, a lady with giant mollusci on the genitals was seen in my department. It was so surprising at that moment to come across such a case. The journey from that very first case has been fascinating. HIV has really opened up the vistas for a skillful clinicians to widen his/her knowledge to a very great extent.

For the last 25 years in my clinical practice, I have seen an absolute rise in number of patients living with HIV/AIDS (PLHA). These patients resent with myriads of mucocutaneous manifestations. At times, it becomes challenge to diagnose the condition, as one may come across atypical presentation of a common disorder. During such times, an idea crossed my mind to compile, whatever material I had, should be utilized. Hence, a comprehensive atlas on HIV-AIDS was conceived.

The atlas is an attempt to provide support to the postgraduate students, general practitioners and young dermatologists to nurture as well as develop a good clinical judgment, so as to be able to pick-up HIV at the earliest.

Bela J Shah

Acknowledgments

I take an opportunity to thank profusely to my postgraduate teacher, mentor and guide, Dr Bharat H Shah, who initiated me into the field of dermatology.

I am indebted to my parents and my husband Ushir and my son Soham, who always felt deprived of quality time, which we could have spent together.

I acknowledge with a deep sense of gratitude, the constant help provided by my postgraduate students Dr Dipti Behl, Dr Kimy Khan, Dr Pooja Choudhari, Dr Santosh Rathod, Dr Dhwani Vakta, Dr Hiral Prajapati and Dr Shyamgovind Rathoriya.

The present work would have been impossible without Dr Kimy Khan, who penned down important text as well as helped me to get all the required pictures from the back-up CDs.

Dr Pooja Choudhari and Dr Santosh Rathod shared their invaluable time with me. I was very lucky to get many 'helping hands' given by Dr Dipti Behl, Dr Shyamgovind Rathoriya, Dr Dhwani Vakta and Dr Hiral Prajapati, at any given time of the day.

Contents

1 Epidemiology of HIV/AIDS

WORLDWIDE AFFECTION OF HIV AND AIDS

Cases of HIV/AIDS have been reported from virtually every country and can be recognized as a global pandemic. By the end of December 2007, the number of people living with HIV/AIDS was 33.2 million (30.6-36.1million), according to the last report of Joint United Nations Program on HIV/AIDS (UNAIDS). Of these approximately 50 percent are females and 2.5 million are children <15 years of age. Worldwide occurrence of the disease has been shown in Figure 1.1.

About 2.5 million new cases of HIV infection, including 420,000 in children <15 years were reported and the global deaths totaled 2.1 million (330,000 children <15 years included). Agewise distribution is illustrated in Table 1.1.

Reductions in the recent trends of HIV incidence globally have been observed. They may reflect natural trends in pandemic as well as results of prevention programs resulting in behavior change. The HIV epidemic has occurred in waves in different parts of the world, each one having different characteristics depending on the demographics of the country and the region involved. Started in United States and shortly thereafter in Western Europe it began in Sub-Saharan Africa, which was particularly devastated by the wave of HIV. Although the region accounts to 10 to 11 percent of world's population, the number of HIV affected people accounts to more than two-thirds of total people living with HIV infection.

In Asia, about 4 to 9 million people were living with HIV, by the end of 2007, national HIV prevalence being highest in South-East Asia(with wide variation in trends amongst countries). However, the population of some countries is so large (e.g. India and China) that even a low percentage of population affected will account to a large number of people with HIV.

Table 1.1: AIDS epidemic, global summary, December 2007

Number of people living with HIV in 2007	Total	33 million [30–36 million]
	Adults	30.8 million [28.2–34.0 million]
	Women	15.5 million [14.2–16.9 million]
	Children <15 years	2.0 million [1.9–2.3 million]
People newly infected with HIV in 2007	Total	2.7 million [2.2–3.2 million]
	Adults	2.3 million [1.9–2.8 million]
	Children <15 years	370,000 [330,000–410,000]
AIDS deaths in 2007	Total	2.0 million [1.8–2.3 million]
	Adults	1.8 million [1.6–2.1 million]
	Children <15 years	270,000 [250,000–290,000]

Encouragingly, HIV prevalence has declined in Myanmar, Cambodia and Thailand. But it continues to increase in Indonesia and Vietnam.

The major population to introduce the disease were men having sex with men. However, now the trend seems to change in developed countries, heterosexuals replacing the homosexuals, followed by IDU's.

Trends and Magnitude of HIV/AIDS in India

India is the second most populous country in the world, with more than 880 million people in 1993. With less than 1 percent of the global land mass, India has more than 16 percent of the world's population, more than that of South America, Africa, and Australia combined. The population will exceed one billion by 2000, surpassing

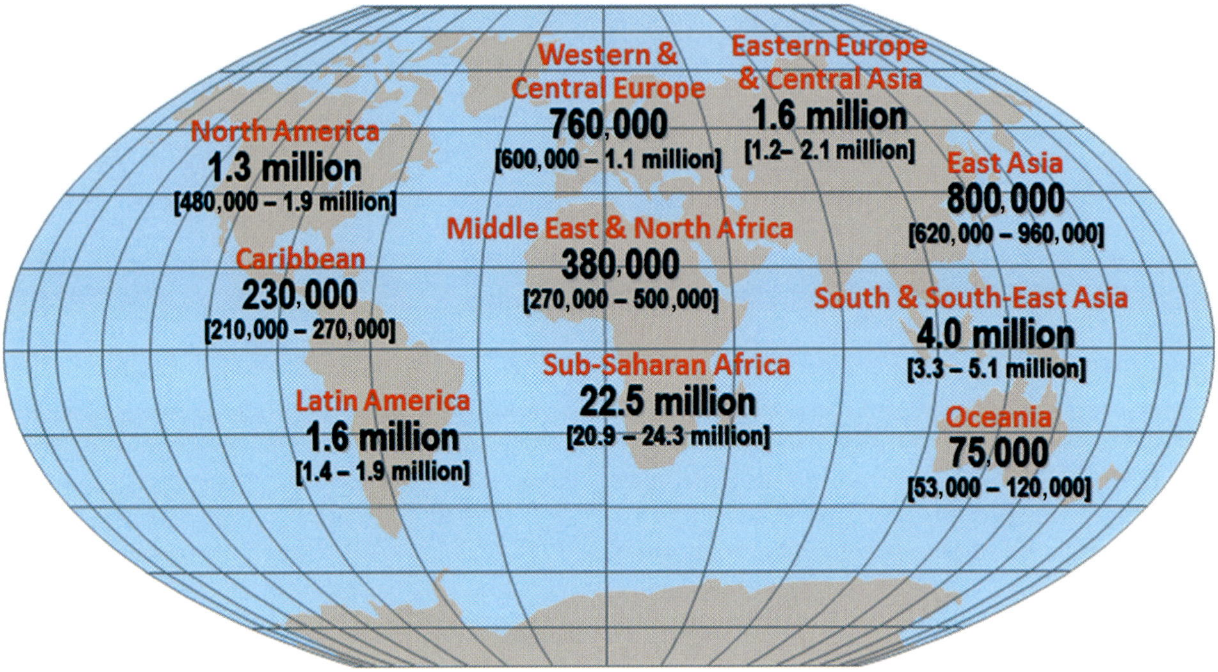

Total: 33 million (30–36 million)

Fig. 1.1: Adults and children living with HIV, December 2007

even China. By then, India will have more new cases of HIV infection per year than any single country, and probably the largest number of HIV-infected people as well. Whatever happens in India will therefore have a major impact upon the global pandemic of HIV and AIDS.

The year 1986 saw first case of HIV infection as well as first report of AIDS case in India. Since then the epidemic has spread throughout the country.

There is an estimated 5.7 million people infected with HIV in India today. The most rapid and well-documented spread of infection has occurred in Mumbai and the State of Tamil Nadu. The infection affects both urban and rural areas. According to the new estimates released by NACO (National AIDS Control Organisation), supported by WHO and UNAIDS, the national HIV prevalence in India is approximately 0.36 percent, which corresponds to about 2 to 3.1 million people living with HIV most cases seen in 15 to 49 years age group (agewise distribution in Table 1.2), signifying the threat of the disease still to the cream part of the society. The highest prevalence rate has been seen in states Maharashtra, Andhra Pradesh and Karnataka in South, Manipur, Mizoram and Nagaland in North East (Fig. 1.2 graphical presentation and Fig. 1.3 pie diagram of Indian states). There are 26 districts with a high prevalence rate, mainly in the states Madhya Pradesh, Uttar Pradesh, West Bengal, Orissa, Rajasthan and Bihar.

Table 1.2: Percentage distribution of people living with HIV/AIDS by age, India, 2006

Age group	*% Distribution*
Adults (15–49 years)	89
Adults (>50 years)	7
Children (<15 years)	4

Source: NACO-HIV sentinel surveillance and HIV estimation, 2006

The HIV and AIDS is increasingly and significantly affecting the young girls and women, especially where heterosexuality is main mode of transmission. Of the adults affected with HIV/AIDS, 39 percent were females.

The HIV epidemic has grown silently in India over the past decade, with the virus spread mainly

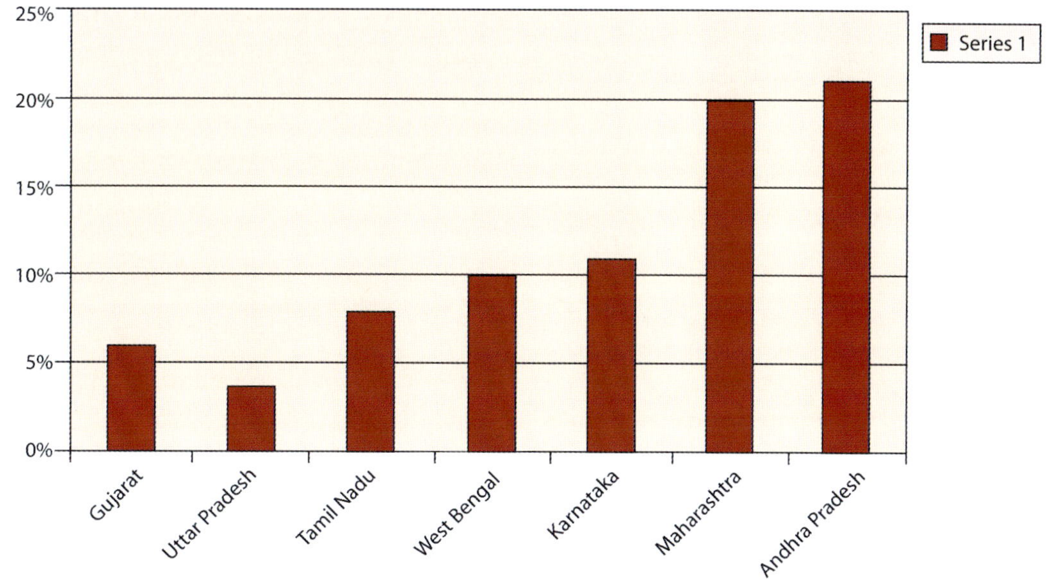

Fig. 1.2: HIV prevalence among different Indian states, India, 2007 (*Source*: HIV sentinel surveillance and HIV estimation 2007)

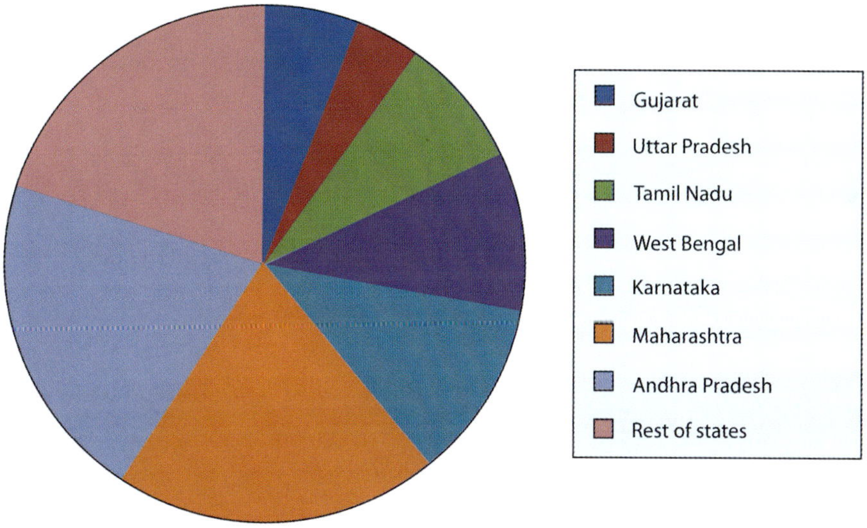

Fig. 1.3: Distribution of PLHA among High Burden States: 2007 (*Source*: HIV sentinel surveillance and HIV estimation 2007)

through heterosexual intercourse. All known routes of transmission are, however, known in India, and increasing seroprevalence has been noted among prostitutes, STD clinic patients, blood donors, and IV drug users. The population has been largely ignorant of the advance of HIV, with public officials and the media at a loss to adequately inform the public about what is taking place. Greater energy and resources are now being devoted to the problem. In the recent years there is evidence of epidemic being stabilized with decrease in new infections reported from some parts of the country.

Molecular Epidemiology

National AIDS Control Programme, phase III is geared to contain the epidemic. HIV viruses circulating in India predominantly belong to HIV-1 subtype C. However, there have been occasional reports of HIV-1 subtype A and B. Matter of concern is reports of A/C and B/C mosaic viruses that are being reported from different parts of the country. The data on HIV drug resistance from India is rather limited. Most of the studies have shown that the virus strains from drug naive patients do not show significant level of drug resistance mutations. The few immunological studies in Indian patients show that the Indian HIV infected patients show both HIV-specific CTL (cytolytic T lymphocytes) responses as well as neutralizing antibody response. Mapping of CTL epitopes showed that while Indian patients identify same regions of gag antigen as recognized by South African subtype C infected patients, some regions are uniquely recognized by Indian patients. There are very few studies on host genetic factors in India in context with HIV infection. However, there are evidences reported of association of host genetic factors such as HLA types and haplotypes and HIV disease.

2 Human Immunodeficiency Virus

AIDS was first identified in United States (Los Angeles) in 1981 in patients with *Pneumocystis jirovecii* (formerly *P. carinii*) pneumonia in five previously healthy homosexual men.

The etiologic agent of AIDS, human immunodeficiency virus (HIV), belongs to the family of human retroviruses (Retroviridae) and the subfamily of lentiviruses. It is a lymphoproliferative retrovirus.

STRUCTURE (FIG. 2.1)

On Electron microscopy, HIV virion is an icosahedral virus containing external spikes formed by the two major envelope proteins, the external gp 120 and the transmembrane gp 41 (Fig. 2.1). The inner cone shaped core encloses the ribonucleoproteins. The genome is diploid, made of two single stranded positive sense RNA

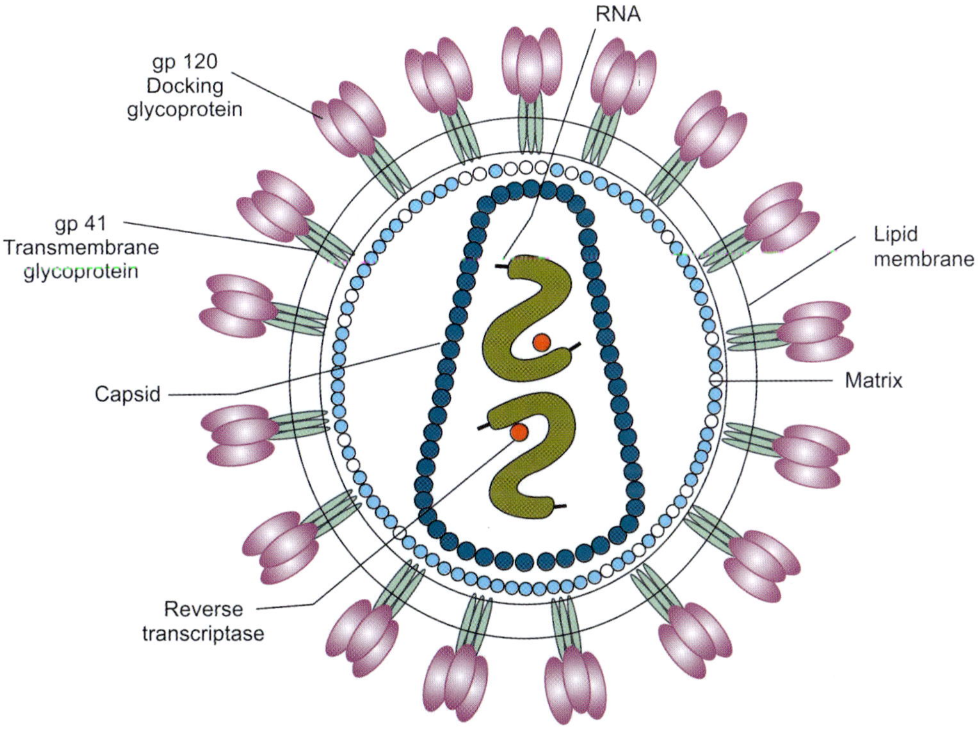

Fig. 2.1: Structure of HIV

copies. During replication when the virion buds from the surface of the infected cell it acquires a lipoprotein envelope consisting of lipids (host cell derived) and glycoprotein (virus coded).

HIV-1 has genes that encode the structural proteins of the virus: *Gag* encodes the proteins forming core of the virion (gp 24, p 18, p 15 antigen); *Pol* encodes the enzymes such as polymerase reverse transcriptase, protease and endonuclease; and *Env* encodes the envelope glycoproteins-gp 160 that cleaves into gp 120 forming outer spikes and gp 41, which is a transmembrane anchoring protein.

There are other nonstructural and regulatory genes (*Tat, Rev, Nef, Vif, Vpr* and *Vpu*), which code for proteins involved in the modification of the host cell to enhance virus growth and the regulation of viral gene expression (Fig. 2.3).

Flanking these genes are the long terminal repeats (LTRs), which contain regulatory elements involved in gene expression. The major difference between the genomes of HIV-1 and HIV-2 is that HIV-2 lacks the *Vpu* gene and has a *Vpx* gene not contained in HIV-1.

Based on antigenic variation HIV-1 is classified as:

- Group M (Major) subtype A to K
- Group O (Outliner)
- Group N (New).

LIFE CYCLE AND PATHOGENESIS

The replication cycle of HIV begins with the binding of the gp 120 protein to its receptor on the host cell surface, the CD4 molecule (Fig. 2.2 EM Presentation). The CD4 molecule is predominantly found on a subset of T lymphocytes responsible for helper function in the immune system. It is also expressed on the surface of monocytes/macrophages and dendritic/Langerhans cells. After binding of gp 120 binds to CD4, the gp 120 undergoes a conformational change that facilitates binding to one of a group of coreceptors. The two major coreceptors for HIV-1 are CCR5 and CXCR4. They belong to the family of seven-transmembrane-domain G protein–coupled cellular receptors, and are important for virus entry into the cell. Following binding of the envelope protein to the CD4 molecule associated with the above-mentioned conformational change in the viral envelope gp 120, fusion with the host cell membrane occurs via the newly exposed gp 41 molecule penetrating the plasma membrane of the target cell and then coiling upon itself to bring the virion and target cell together. Following fusion, the entire complex, composed of viral RNA and viral enzymes and surrounded by a capsid protein coat, is released into the cytoplasm of the target cell. When this complex reaches

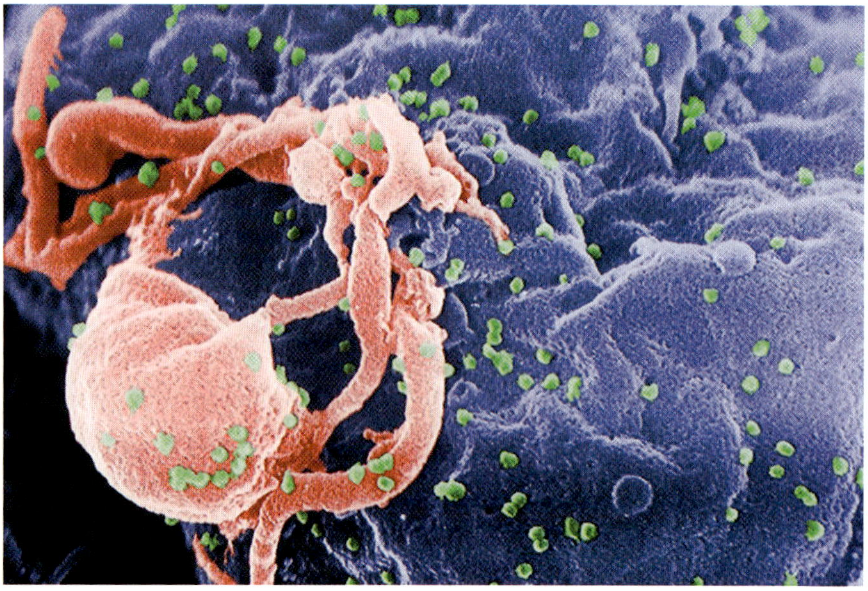

Fig. 2.2: Scanning electron micrograph of HIV-1 budding from cultured lymphocyte. This image has been colored to highlight important features. Multiple round bumps on cell surface represent sites of assembly and budding of virions

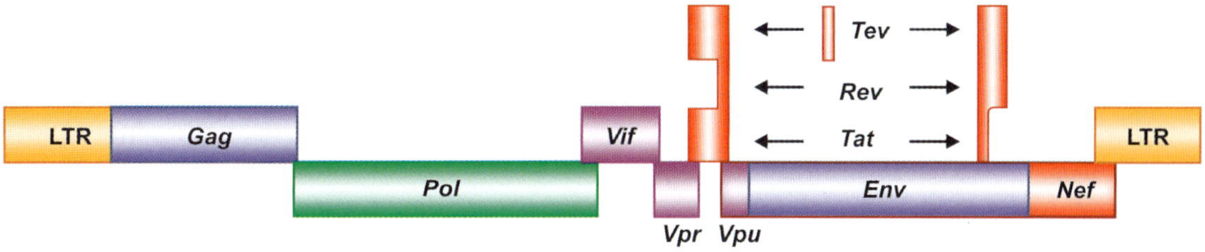

Fig. 2.3: Genomic structure

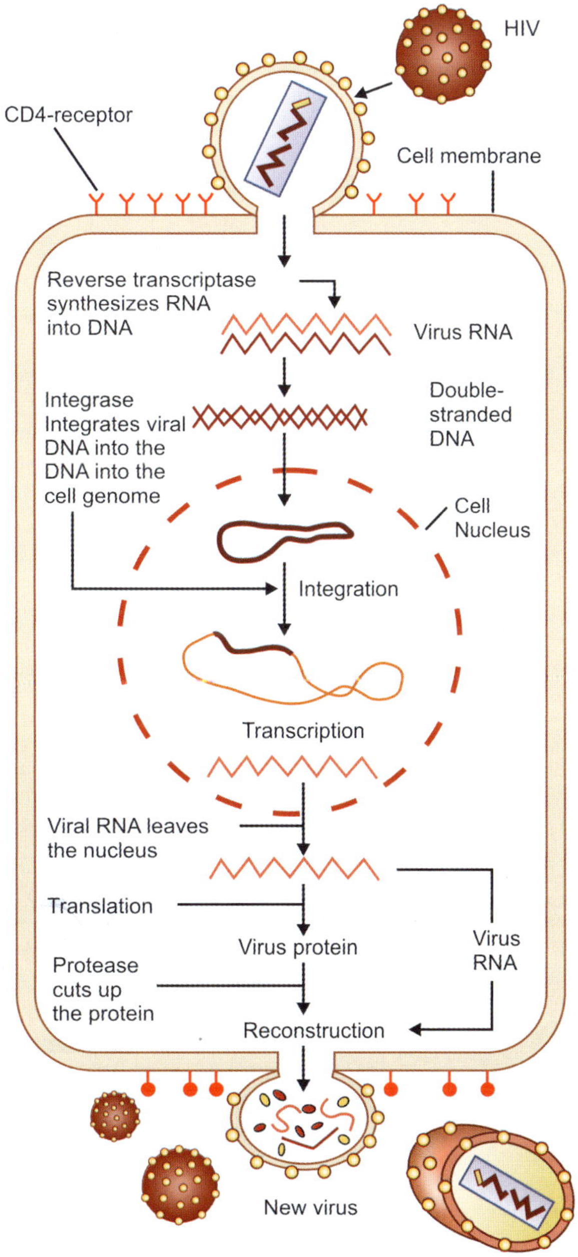

Fig. 2.4: Life cycle of HIV

the nucleus, the viral reverse transcriptase enzyme catalyzes the reverse transcription of the genomic RNA into DNA, and the protein coat opens to release the resulting double-stranded HIV-DNA (Fig. 2.4).

The hallmark of HIV disease is immunodeficiency resulting primarily from a progressive quantitative and qualitative deficiency of the helper T-cells, which contain on it's surface, the CD4 molecule. This CD4 molecule serves as the primary cellular receptor for HIV. Presence of a coreceptor is a must for efficient fusion and entry of HIV-1 into its target cells. These coreceptors (CCR5 and CXCR4) are also the primary receptors for certain chemoattractive cytokines termed *chemokines*.

Various mechanisms responsible for cellular depletion, immune dysfunction and propagation of HIV have been suggestive. These include:

- Direct infection and destruction of these cells by HIV and immune clearance of infected cells
- Indirect effects such as immune exhaustion due to aberrant cellular activation and activation-induced cell death
- Destruction of lymphoid tissue resulting in severe impairment of immune response.

3 Mucocutaneous Infections in HIV/AIDS

Rare diseases and unusual presentations of common diseases, both, are seen by medical personnels, particularly dermatologists.

Infections are the largest category of cutaneous disorders in patients with HIV/AIDS. These infections cover both, those seen in immunocompetent patients as well as the ones seen exclusively in people living with HIV/AIDS (PLHA).

Skin infections in PLHA may present as ususal or with atypical manifestations. Atypical presentation may be due to:

- Decreased immune response in PLHA(especially CD4 positive T cell mediated)
- Infection with more than one organism concurrently.

Mucocutaneous lesions in setting of HIV may be less inflammed than usual, more widespread, more disfiguring or more destructive.

Commonly used classification of mucocutaneous infections is given in Table 3.1.

Table 3.1: Infections and infestations

1. **Viral**
   - Herpes simplex virus
   - Varicella zoster virus
   - Cytomegalo virus
   - Epstein-Barr virus
   - Molluscum contagiosum virus
   - Human papilloma virus
   - Hepatitis B and C virus
   - Human herpes virus 8/Kaposi's sarcoma virus
   - Other viruses—Parvo B 19
2. **Bacterial**
   - *Staphylococcus aureus* infection
   - Bacillary angiomatosis
   - Mycobacterial infections
     - Mycobacterium tuberculosis
     - *Mycobacterium leprae*
     - Atypical mycobacteria (mainly MAIC)
   - Venereal diseases
     - Syphilis
     - Chancroid
     - Granuloma inguinale
     - Lymphogranuloma venereum
     - Gonorrhea
3. **Fungal**
   - Superficial fungal infections
     - Dermatophytosis
     - Candidiasis
     - Pityrosporum infection
   - Deep fungal infections
     - Cryptococcosis
     - Histoplasmosis
     - Coccidiomycosis
     - Aspergillosis
     - *Pneumocystis jirovecii*
     - *Penicillium marneffei*

Contd...

VIRAL INFECTIONS

Viruses are common pathogens producing disease in PLHA. They are one of the major pathogens causing opportunistic infections (OIs) in PLHA. Sometimes mixed infections due to more than one pathogen are seen Fig. 3.25.

Clinical appearance of viral infections in some patients has high predictive value for HIV infection. High-risk patients should be counseled for HIV serology testing if they present with giant mollusci, florid warts (genital or extra genital), hemorrhagic or necrotic herpetic lesions, disseminated or multidermatomal herpes zoster.

Contd...

- Other reported paracoccidiomycosis
  - Blastomycosis
  - Cutaneous sporotrichosis

4. Parasitic
- Scabies
- Leishmaniasis
- Demodicidosis

Some viral infections like herpes simplex increases the transmission and replication of the HIV virus reducing life span of a person with PLHA.

The gene protein of the HIV alter the activity of E6 and E7 proto-oncogenes and therefore predisposes to increased carcinogenic risk.

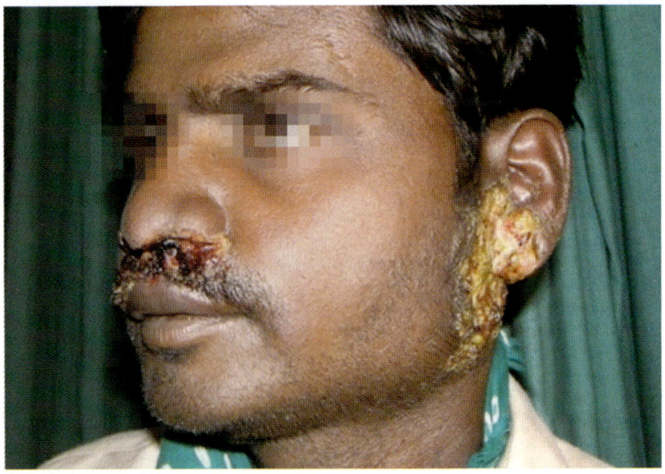

Fig. 3.2: Herpes labialis with vesicles extending to vestibule of nose and preauricular area

Herpes Simplex Infection

The spectrum of clinical manifestations in PLHA includes, hereps simplex virus most commonly presents as genital herpes, other presentations are herpes labialis (Figs 3.1 and 3.2), chronic herpetic ulcers (Figs 3.3 and 3.4) (associated with herpetic colitis), orofacial herpes (Fig. 3.5), herpetic whitlow and herpetic folliculitis (follicular facial lesions).

The presentation of lesions in PLHA may be seen in exaggerated form like pseudotumor tongue, deep ulcers, ecthyma like lesions and systemic involvement

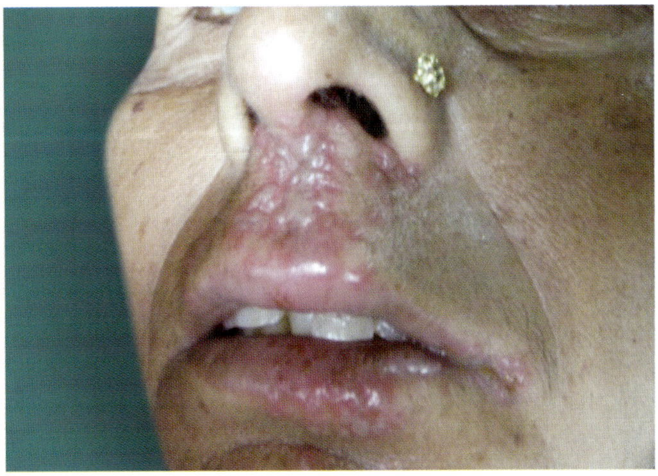

Fig. 3.1: Herpes simplex

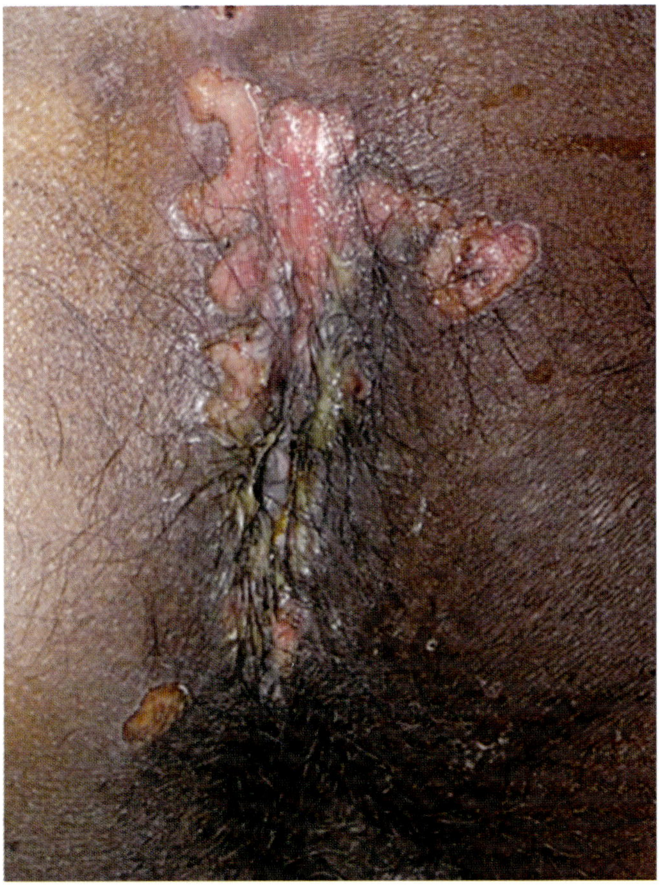

Fig. 3.3: Herpes genitalis (perianal region)

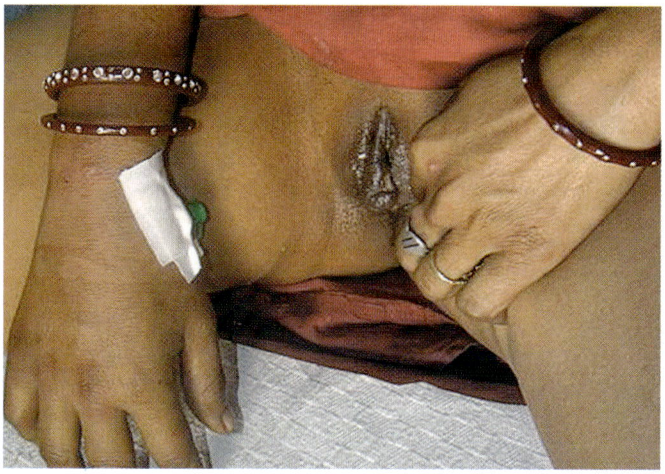

Fig. 3.4: Herpes progenitalis (HSV II) with erythema multiforme

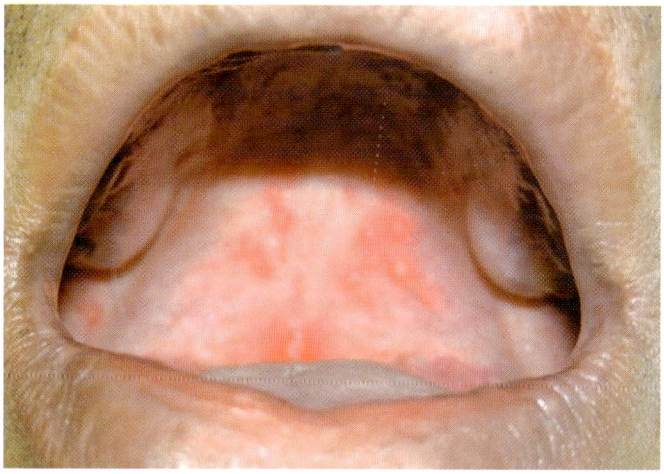

Fig. 3.5: Herpetic aphthous ulcers

like esophagitis, hepatitis, encephalitis, etc. in comparision to immunocompetent hosts. Presence of mucocutaneous HSV infection for more than one month is suggestive of advanced HIV infection.

Treatment remains same as that in immunocompetent patients, i.e. acyclovir 200 mg five times a day, which can be extended in duration. Valacyclovir, famcyclovir are alternatives of acyclovir. However, resistant cases can be offered intravenous foscarnet or cidofovir. Topical cidofovir gel and imiquimod 5 percent and resiquimod is also available for resistant HSV infection.

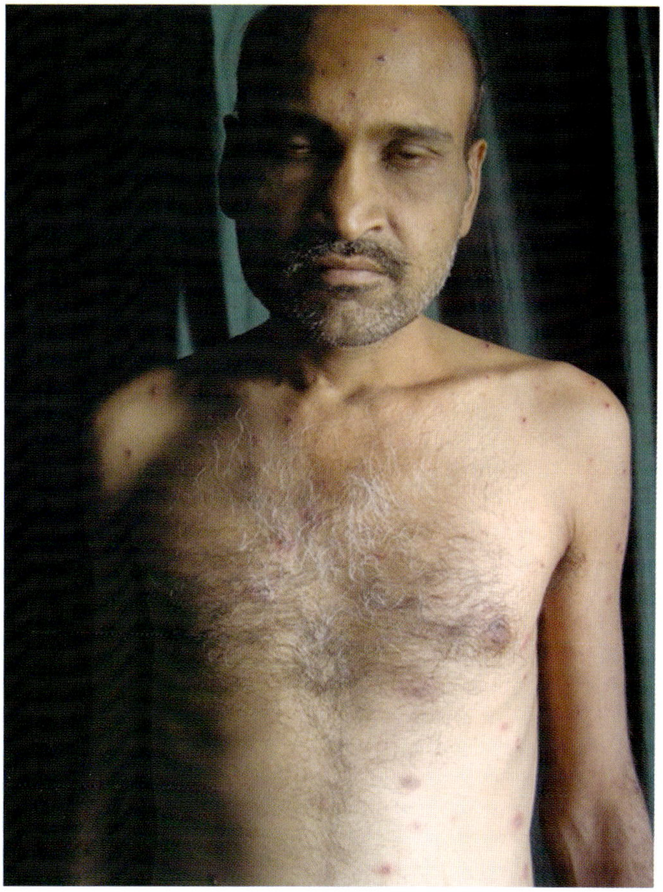

Fig. 3.6: Chickenpox (primary zoster infection)

Treatment resistance is common in HIV positive patients because of thymidine kinase mutations and mutations of DNA polymerase.

These patients may respond to very higher doses of acyclovir or they need drug like foscarnet or cidofovir.

Varicella Zoster Virus

HIV infected patients may develop primary varicella infection (Chickenpox Fig. 3.6) on first exposure or as herpes zoster (Figs 3.9 and 3.10). Course is usually prolonged and complicated (Fig. 3.8) (disseminated as pneumonia, hepatitis, encephalitis or superinfected with bacteria). Lesions of zoster may be uni or multidermatomal (Fig. 3.7) or disseminated in immunocompromised patients. Disseminated zoster can be classified as > 1 non contagious, > 2 contagious

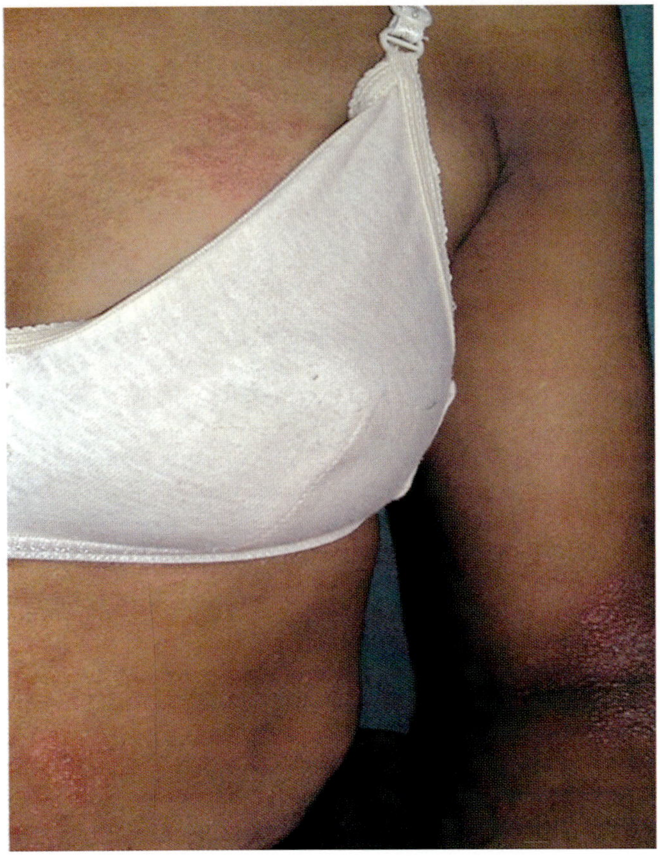

Fig. 3.7: Multidermatomal herpes zoster

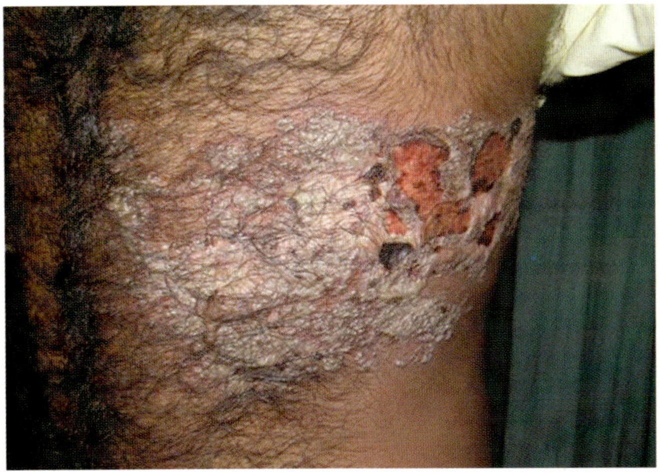

Fig. 3.8: Herpes zoster with ulceration

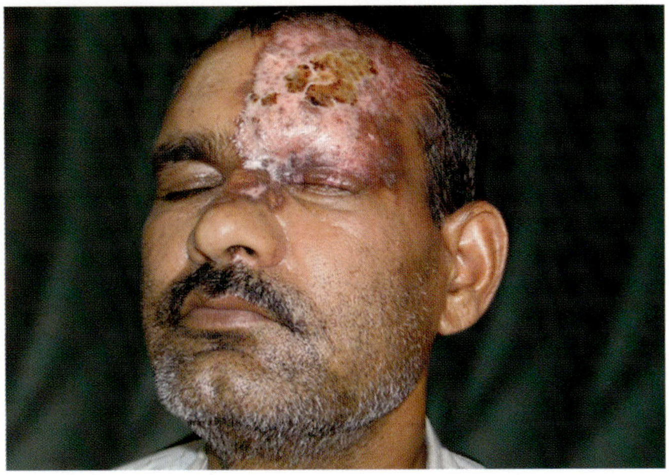

Fig. 3.9: Herpes zoster ophthalmicus

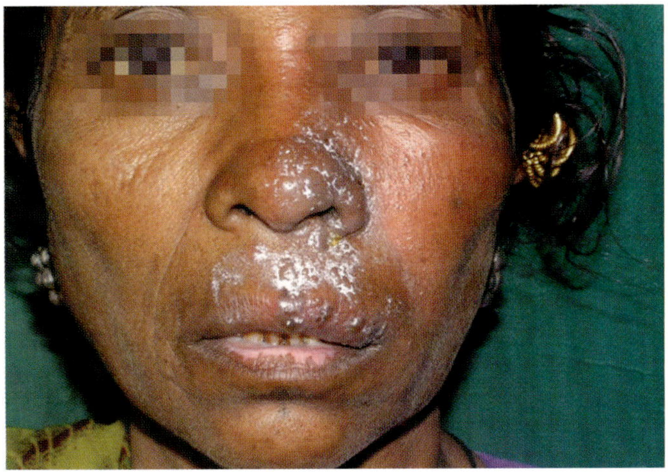

Fig. 3.10: Herpes zoster with mandibular-maxillary division of trigeminal nerve

sites, >20 discrete lesions or systemic involvement. Herpes zoster occurring as IRIS is mild and presents with few lesons but rarely can be disseminated. Neurologic and ophthalmologic (Fig. 3.9) complications are seen. Hutchinson's sign : If tip of nose is involved then neurological involvement is common.

Treatment includes acyclovir 800 mg five times a day for ten or more days or valacyclovir, famcyclovir can be given. In complicated cases, intravenous acyclovir

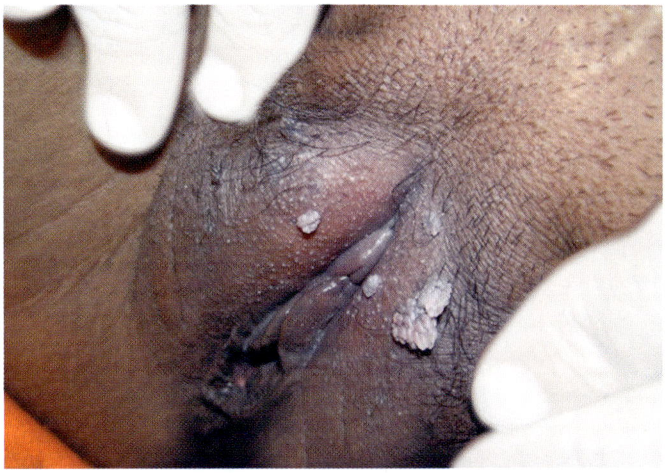

Fig. 3.11: Condyloma acuminata

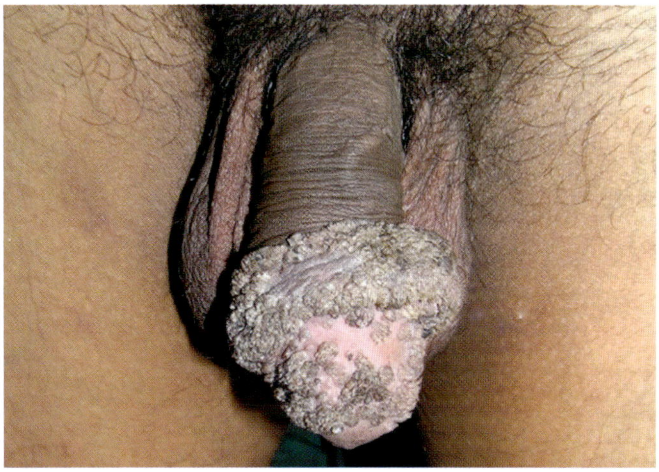

Fig. 3.13: Condyloma acuminata-Keratoic variety

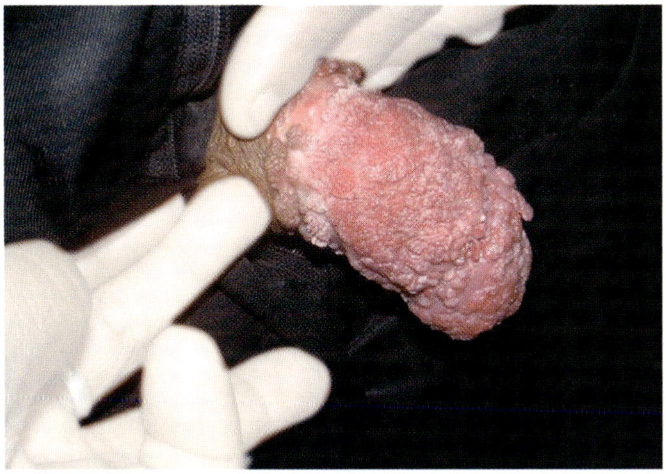

Fig. 3.12: Condyloma acuminata (vascular)

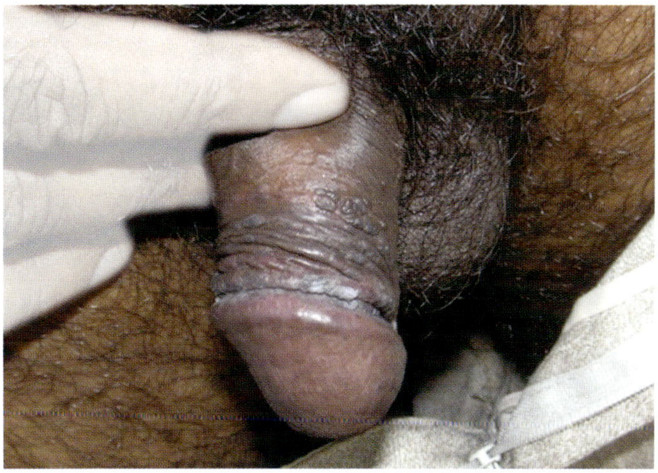

Fig. 3.14: Bowenoid papulosis

(10 mg/kg eight hourly) can be given. Resistant cases are helped by intravenous foscarnet (40 mg/kg every 8 hourly for 10-42 days). Systemic steroids are contraindicated.

Human Papilloma Virus

Prevalence of verruca plana (Fig. 3.18) as well as vulgaris (Figs 3.17, 3.19 to 3.21) is increasing in PLHA. Lesions are much more florid (Figs 3.15A and B) and unresponsive to treatment. HIV infected patients have higher rates of cancers associated with HPV infection. HPV is also known to cause Bowenoid papulosis (Fig. 3.14), hyperpigmented papules with flat surface present over genitalia. Condyloma acuminata (Figs 3.11 to 3.13) seen over genitals, rarely it may increase in size and such giant acuminata are reffered as Bushcke Lowenstein tumor, which is a squamous cell carcinoma *in situ*.

Treatment (Figs 3.15A and B) include topical modalities mainly i.e. cryosurgery, electrosurgery, 20% podopyllin, imiquimod intralesional bleomycin, intralesional interferons.

HPV vaccine (recombinant) made from L1, L2 genes is also available, which is mainly active against type 6, 11, 16, 18. Dosage at 0, 2, 6 or 8 weeks for prophylaxis in adolescent girls.

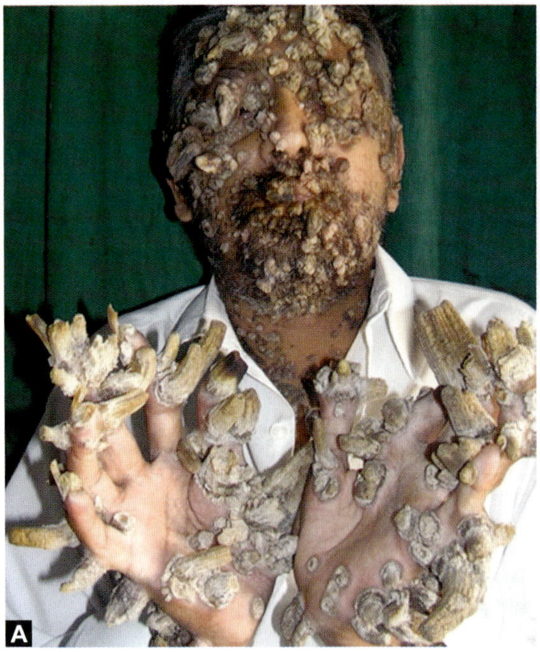
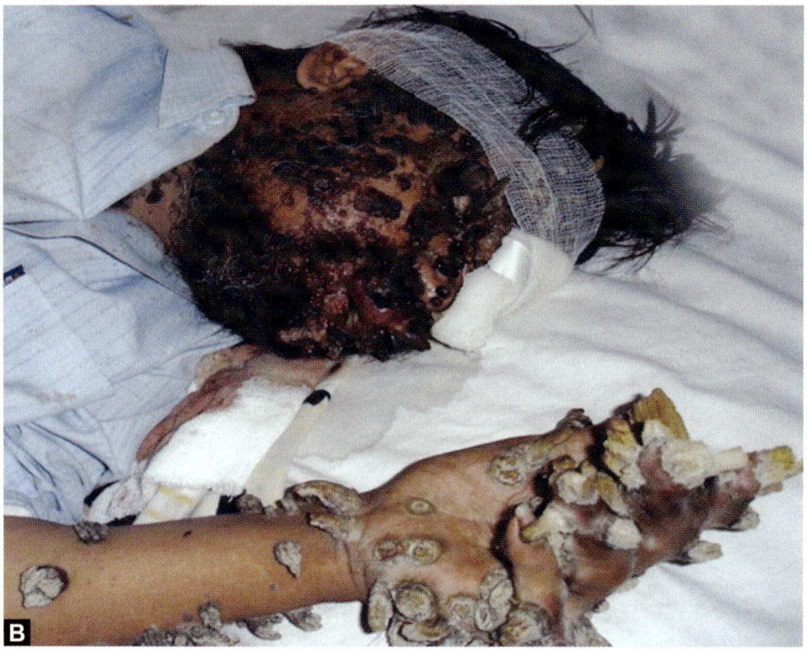

Figs 3.15A and B: (A) Horny changes over cutaneous; (B) Warts

Oral Hairy Leukoplakia (OHL)

A presumptive diagnosis of the condition can be made clinically, but, EBV should be identified to assign this diagnosis. It does not predispose to malignancy as in other leukoplakias.

Treatment is rarely indicated for, as it is a benign condition and usually disappears with commencement of ART (Figs 3.16A and B). High dose of acyclovir and ganciclovir has been proposed.

Molluscum Contagiosum Virus

This infection is most common with dramatic reduction in immune function of the HIV infected individual. Papules can be multiple (Fig. 3.25), tiny, giant (>2 cm) (Fig. 3.23) and atypical (Figs 3.22 and 3.24).

However, there are various other mimickers like cryptococcosis, histoplasmosis, penicilliosis, so the diagnosis for a giant papule with umbilication needs to be confirmed by biopsy, etc. differential diagnosis includes cryptococcosis, penicilliosis, histoplasmosis, etc. Tiny and atypical molluscum may mimick comedones, acne, syringomas, keratoacanthomas, basal cell carcinomas, ecthyma, cutaneous horn, etc.

BACTERIAL INFECTIONS

Staphylococcus aureus is the most common bacterial pathogen in HIV infected persons. Common infections include impetigo, furuncles (Figs 3.26 and 3.28), carbuncles, ecthyma, folliculitis (Figs 3.27, 3.29 to 3.31), cellulitis, etc.

Treatment is identical to that in immunocompetent patients. Rifampicin, 600 mg daily for five to ten days, can be given in recurrent and non responsive infections.

Tuberculosis is the most common opportunistic infection in PLHA patients in India. Treatment guidelines are same as that in non HIV infected patients.

Type of cutaneous tuberculosis includes lupus Vulgaris (Fig. 3.36), tuberculosis verrucosa cutis, scrofuloderma, (Figs 3.40A and B) milliary tuberculosis, tuberculous lymphadenitis, papulonecrotic tuberculides (Figs 3.37 to 3.39).

Biopsy of lesion may cause difficulty in diagnosis due to absence of typical granuloma because of a decrease in CMI of the patients.

Atypical mycobacteria MAC (*Mycobacterium avium* complex) usually causes skin lesions that presents as multiple papules (Figs 3.42 to 3.44), nodules, (Fig. 3.39) ulceration.

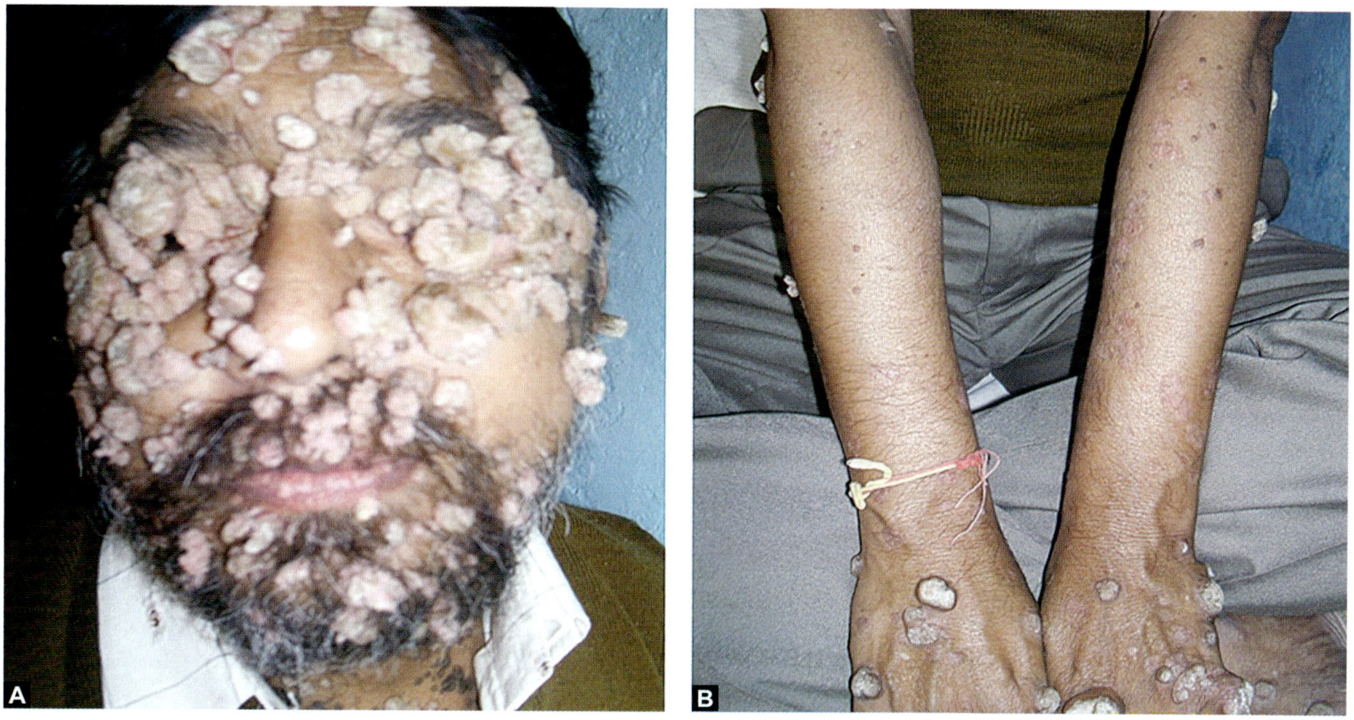

Figs 3.16A and B: Response of ART and immunomodulators in cutaneous warts (follow-up of the patient in Figs 3.15A and B)

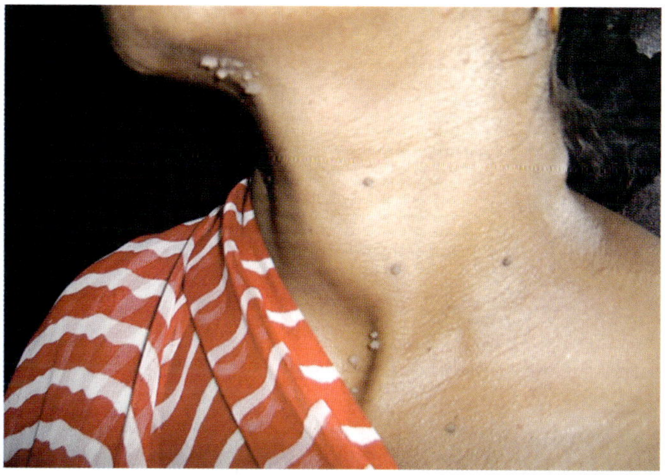

Fig. 3.17: Verruca vulgaris

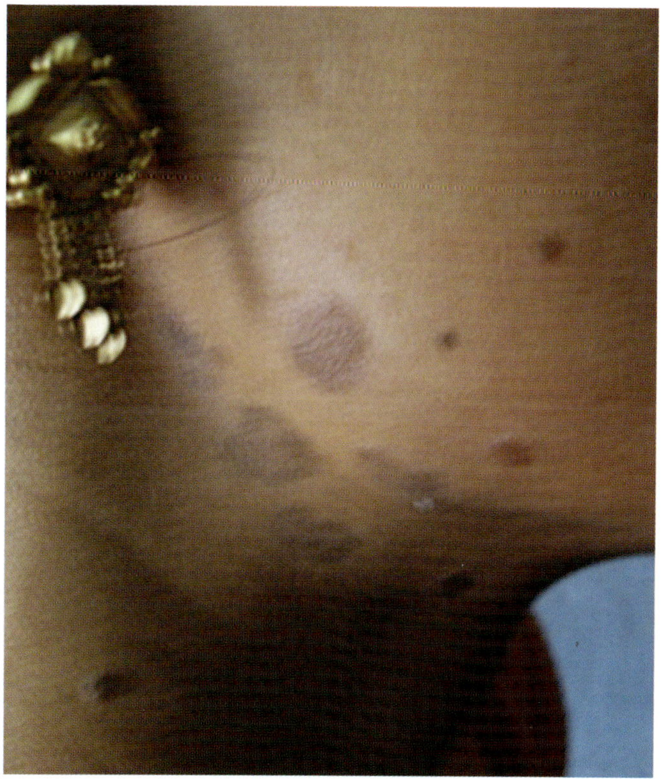

Fig. 3.18: Verruca plana

Bacillary angiomatosis: It is caused by *Bartonella henselae* and rarely by *Bartonella quintana*.

In HIV positive patients, the infection present as multiple angioproliferative lesions on skin, mucosa and internal organs.Tiny pinpoint papules resembling cherry angiomas are present widely in large numbers

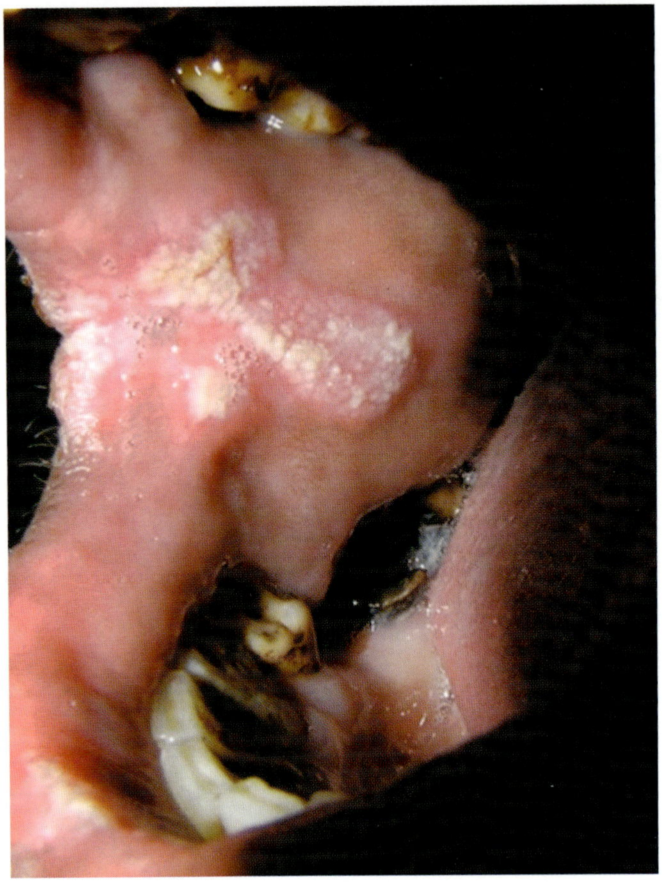
Fig. 3.19: Oral (mucosal) wart

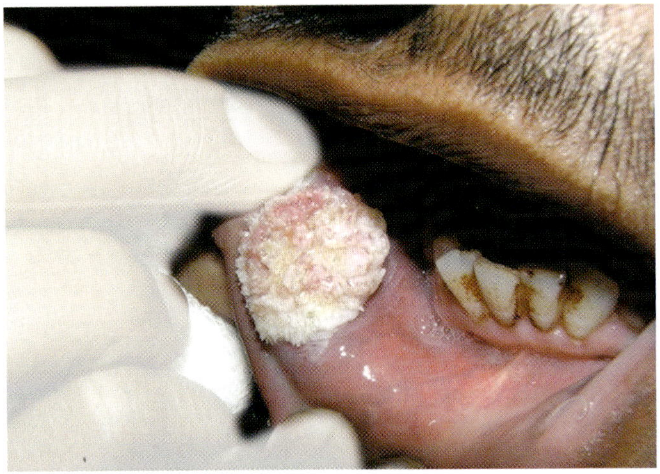
Fig. 3.20: Verruca vulgaris in oral cavity

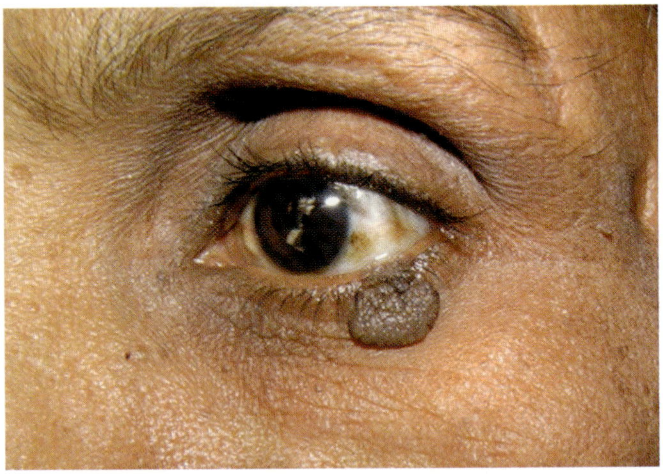
Fig. 3.21: Wart present over inferior eyelid margin

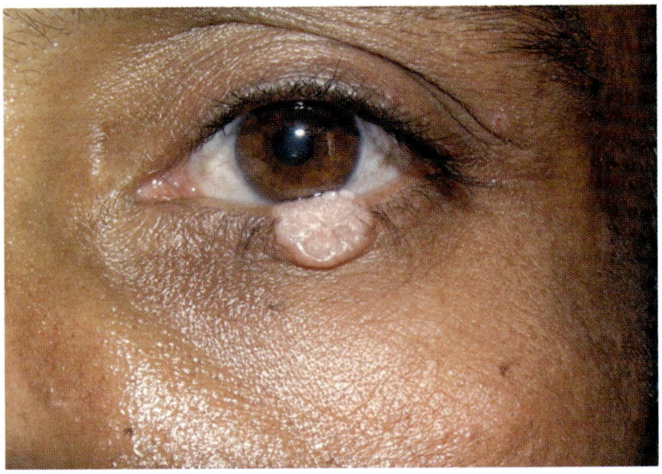
Fig. 3.22: Molluscum contagiosum over lower eyelid

and enlarge rapidly. Identification can be done by using Warthin starry stain, which is specific for this bacillus.

Treatment includes erythromycin (500 mg) QID for 3–4 weeks or doxycycline (100 mg) 1 bd for 3–4 weeks.

Cutaneous malakoplakia is a rare ,chronic,infectious condition that is characterized by granulomatous inflammation primarily in immunocompromised host (Figs 3.32 and 3.33).

Increased prevalence and atypical presentation of leprosy has been found in HIV (Figs 3.41A and B)

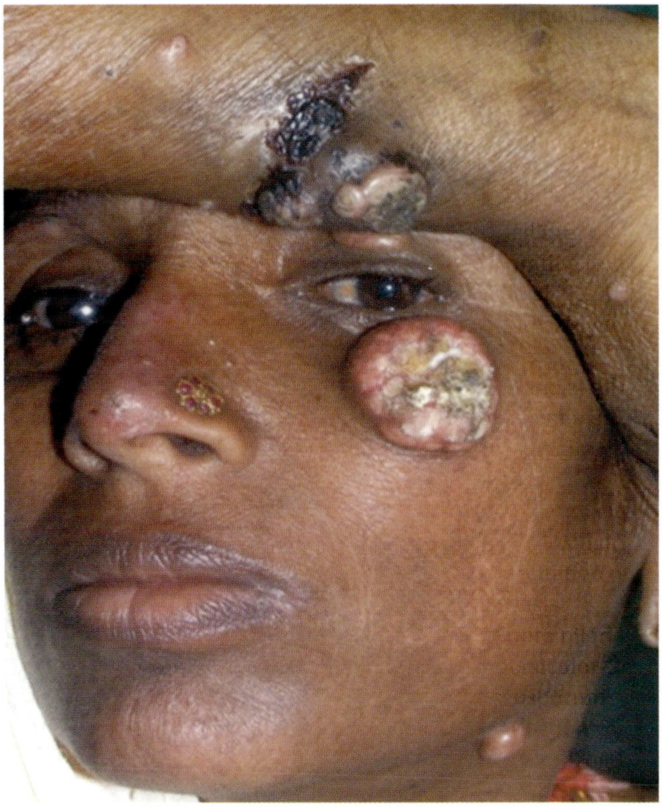

Fig. 3.23: Giant molluscum on face, hand with infection and ulceration on hand

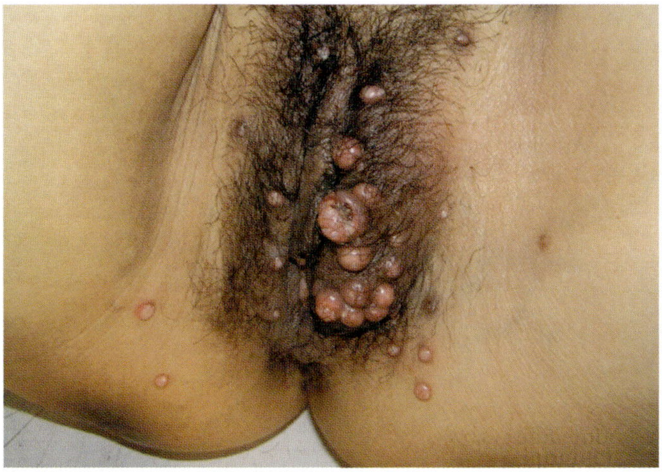

Fig. 3.24: Molluscum contagiosum with giant and inflammed lesions

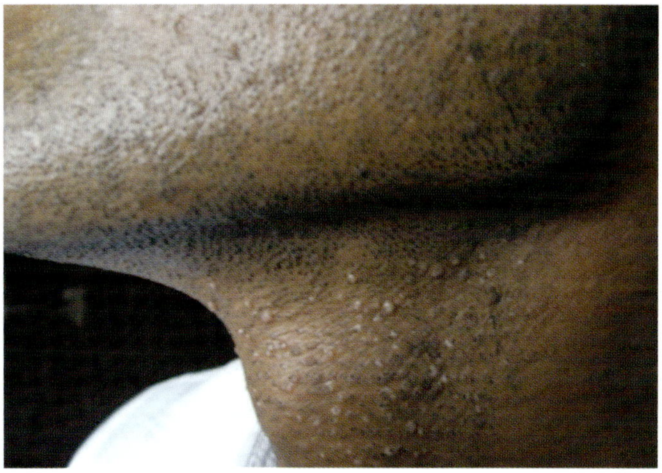

Fig. 3.25: Verruca plana along with molluscum contagiosum

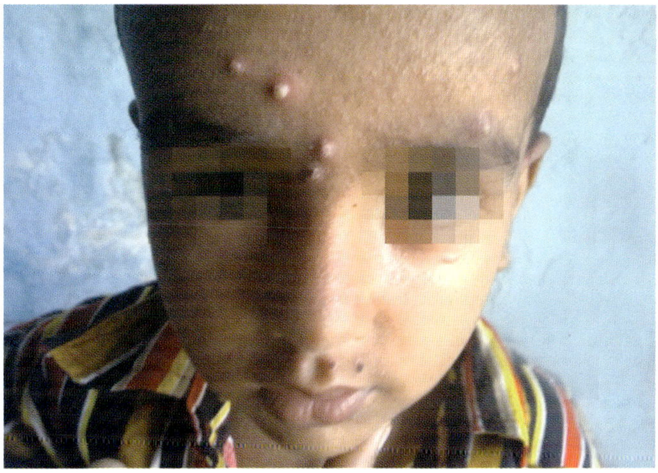

Fig. 3.26: Furuncles

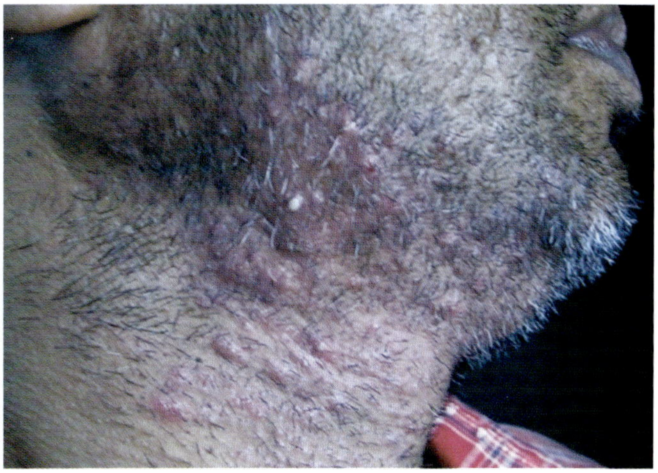

Fig. 3.27: Sycosis barbae

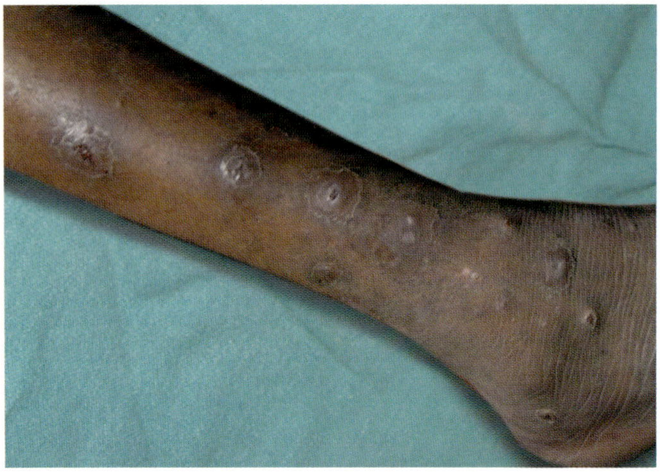

Fig. 3.28: Multiple furuncles over lower leg

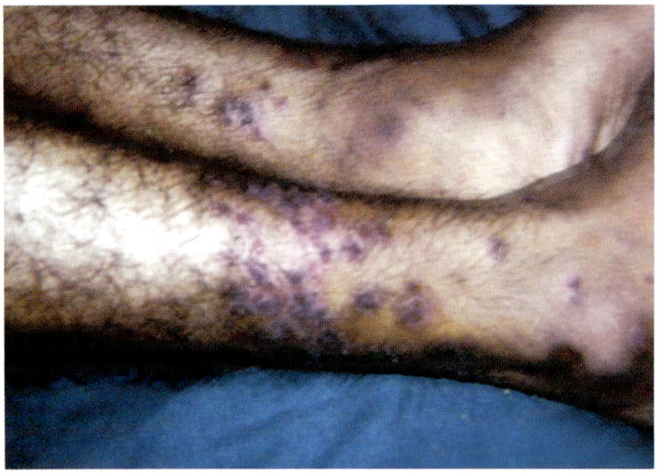

Fig. 3.29: Chronic folliculitis over lower legs

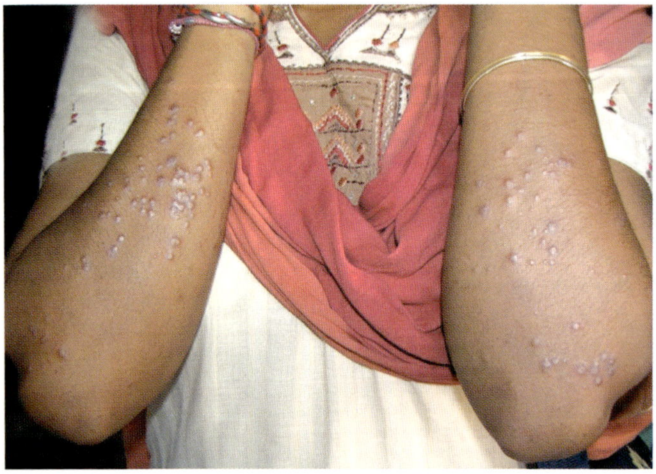

Fig. 3.30: Folliculitis

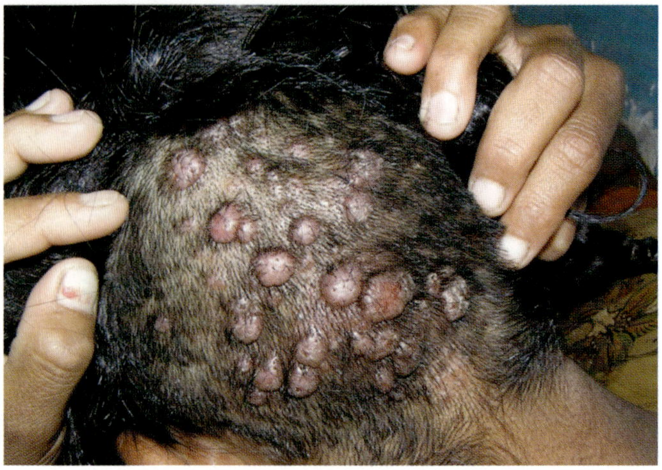

Fig. 3.31: Botryomycosis

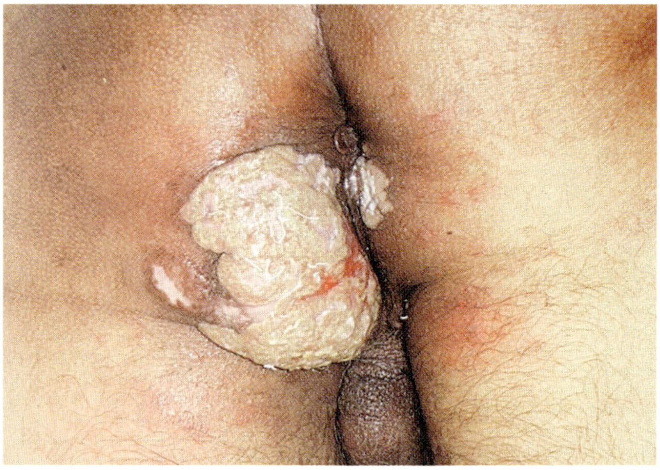

Fig. 3.32: Malakoplakia

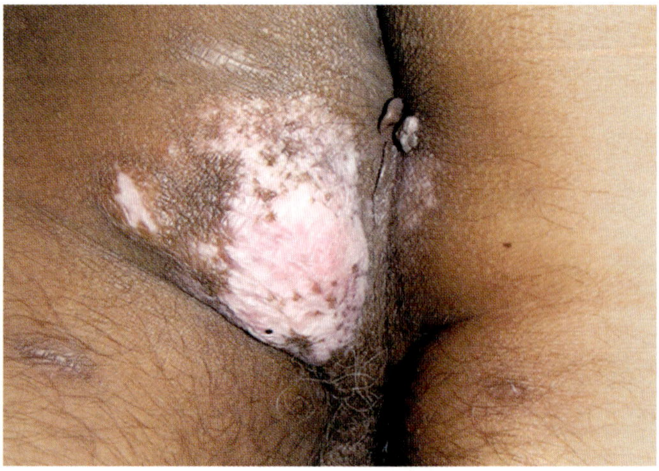

Fig. 3.33: Malakoplakia after treatment with tinidazole

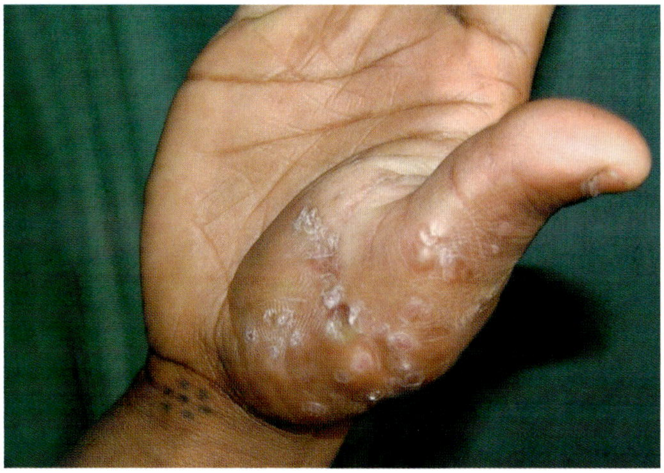

Fig. 3.34: Actinomycosis—woody edema with multiple erythematous papules and draining sinuses over the thenar eminence and the dorsal aspect of right thumb

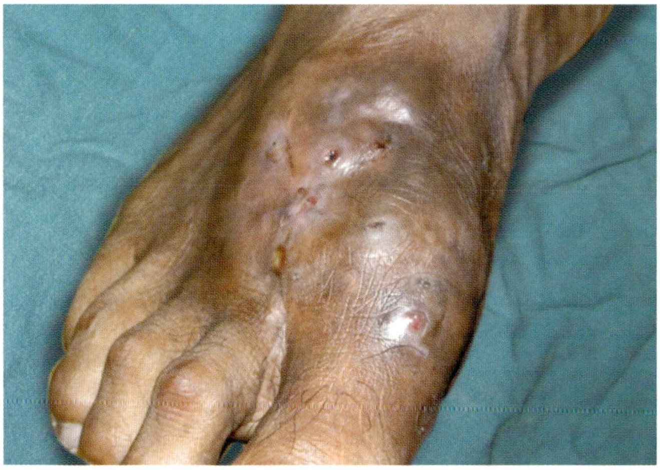

Fig. 3.35: Mycetoma foot—multiple draining sinuses and nodules the dorsum of the foot discharging granules

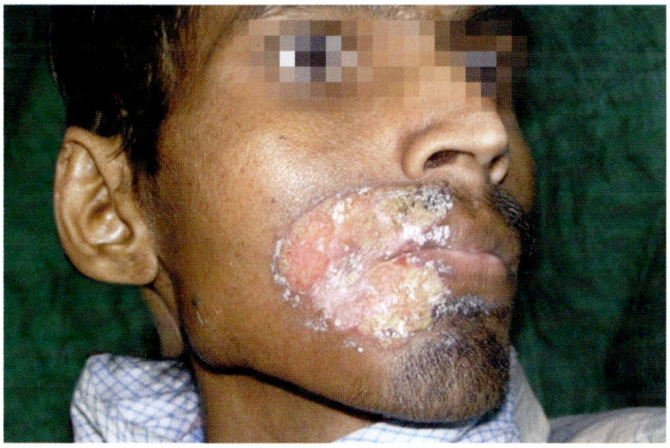

Fig. 3.36: Lupus vulgaris

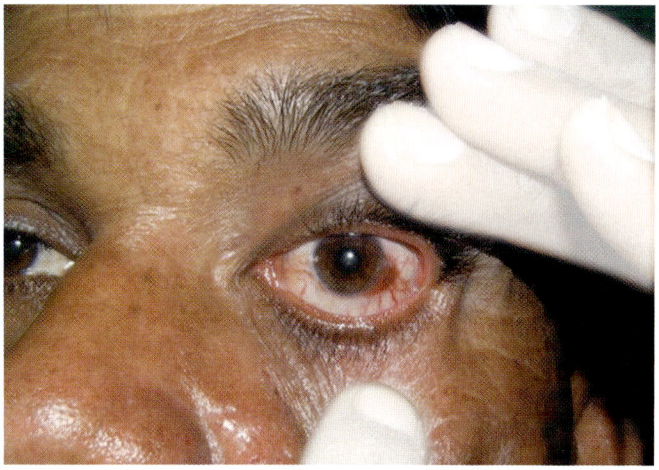

Fig. 3.37: Phlyctenular conjunctivitis

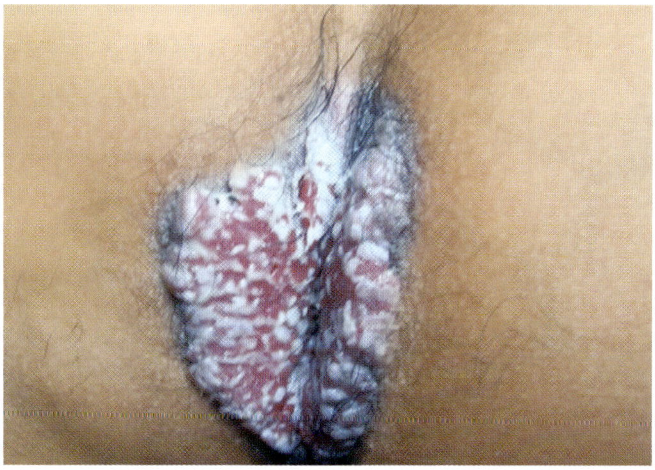

Fig. 3.38: Periorificial tuberculosis

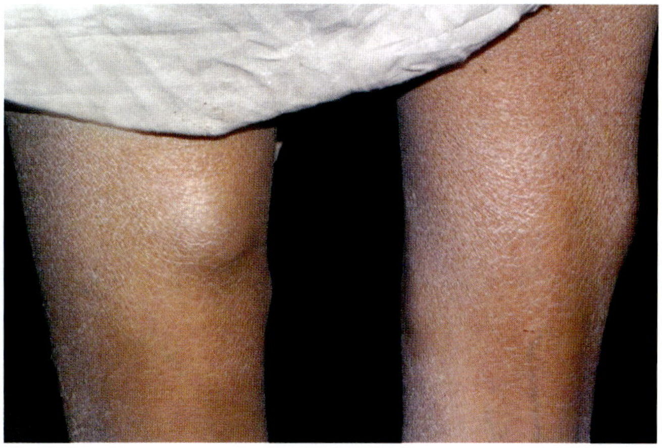

Fig. 3.39: Subcutaneous nodules (tuberculous) with xerosis

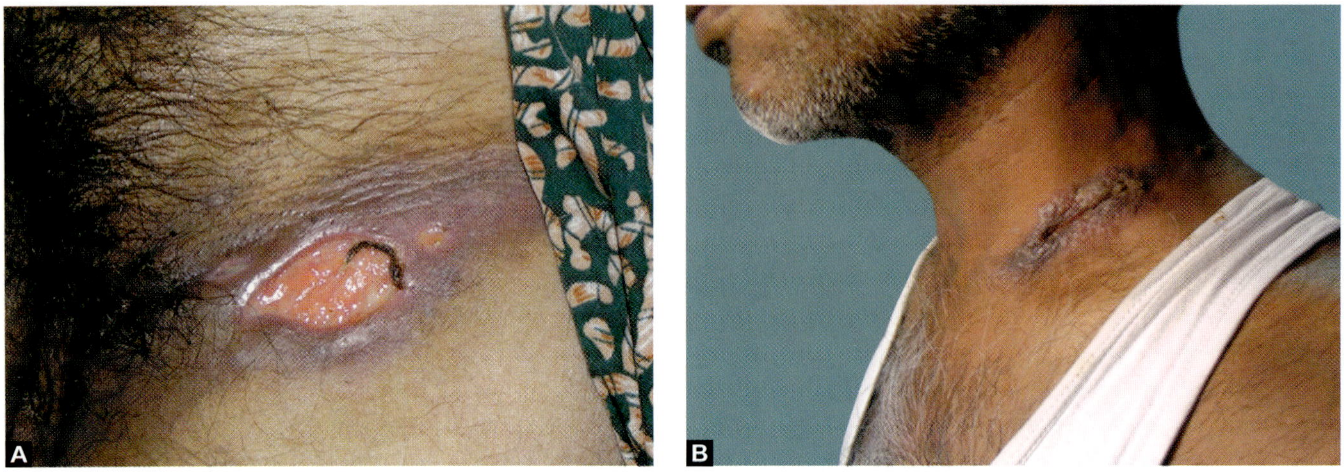

Figs 3.40A and B: Scrofuloderma

MYCOBACTERIAL INFECTIONS

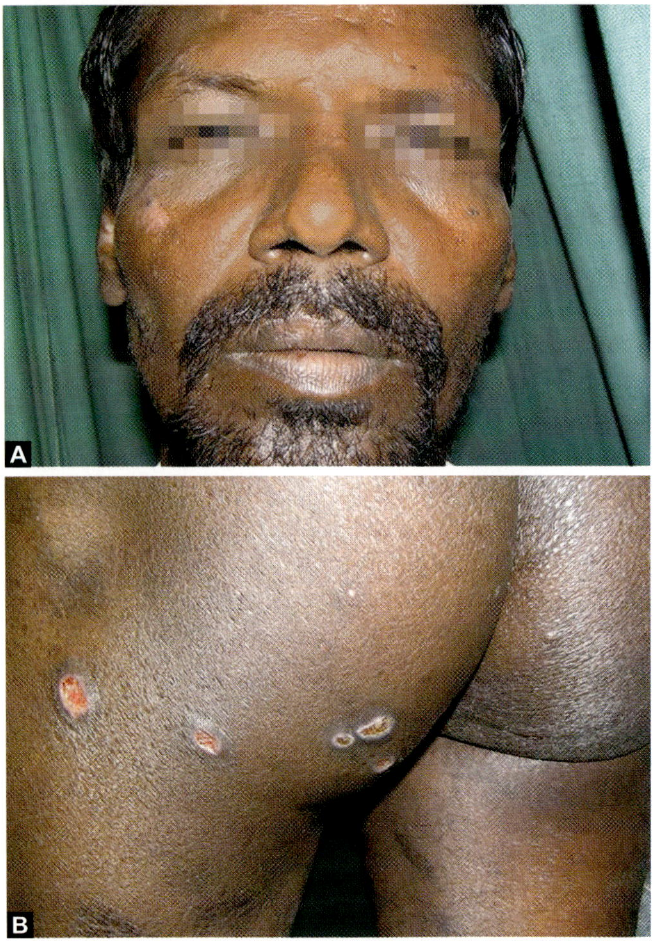

Figs 3.41A and B: (A) Diffuse infiltration on the face; (B) Leprosy with vasculitic ulcers over buttock

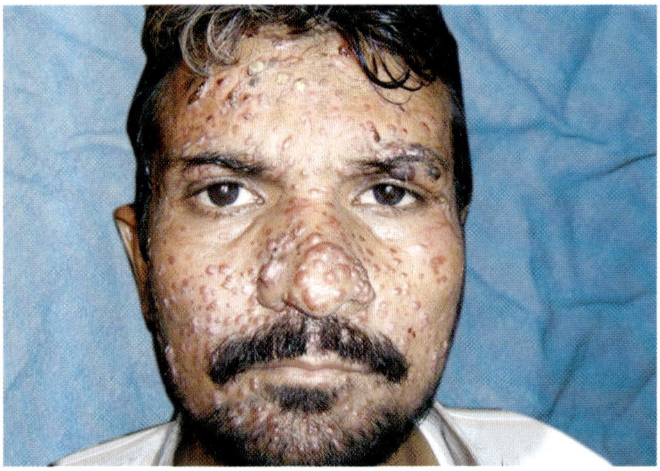

Fig. 3.42: Atypical mycobacterial infection presenting with papulonodular lesions on face

FUNGAL INFECTIONS

This class of infections can present with superficial or deep mycosis (Figs 3.32 to 3.35).

Cadidiasis (Fig. 3.46) can affect oral mucosa (atrophic, hyperplastic, angular cheilitis), esophagus or vulvovaginal mucosa. Systemic antifungals are advocated as topical antifungals give transient relief. Fluconazole 100–200 mg for 10–14 days is preferred regimen. Fluconazole refractory cases can be managed with itraconazole or amphotericin B or even voriconazole.

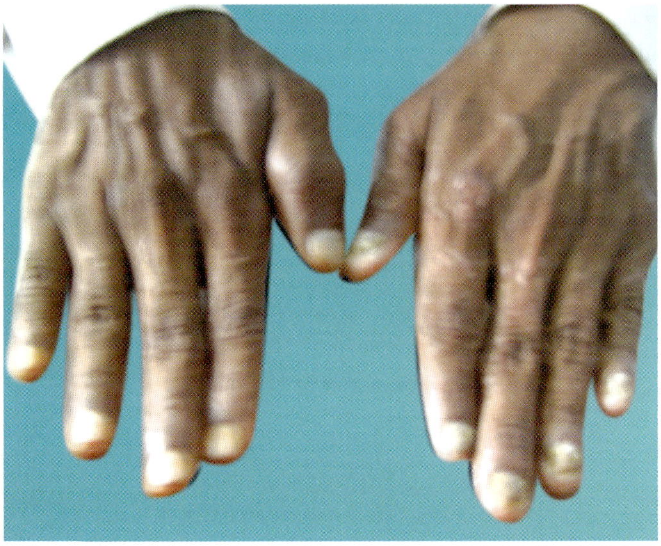

Fig. 3.43: Dorsum of hands of the same patient with few lesions seen over left hand along with onychomycosis

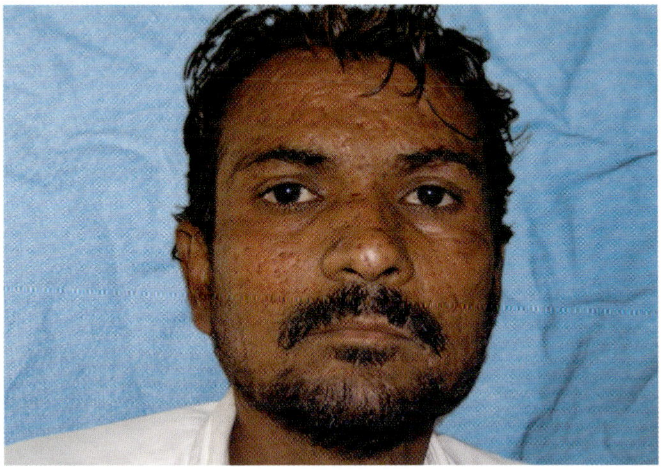

Fig. 3.44: Follow-up of the patient in Fig 3.44 with resolution of lesions after treating with clarithromycin and doxycyline for 8 weeks

Tinea (Figs 3.48 and 3.49) is most commonly caused by ***Trichophyton rubrum*** fungus. Onychomycosis (Fig. 3.47) seen as proximal superficial white onychomycos is characteristic of HIV infection. Total dystrophic onychomycosis may also be seen. Oral and/or systemic antifungals are used, like, fluconazole and itraconazole in addition topical antifungal. Oropharyngeal candidiasis causing dysphagia may present as creamy white cottage cheese (pseudomembranous) like plaques on tongue, palate, buccal mucosa and tonsils or

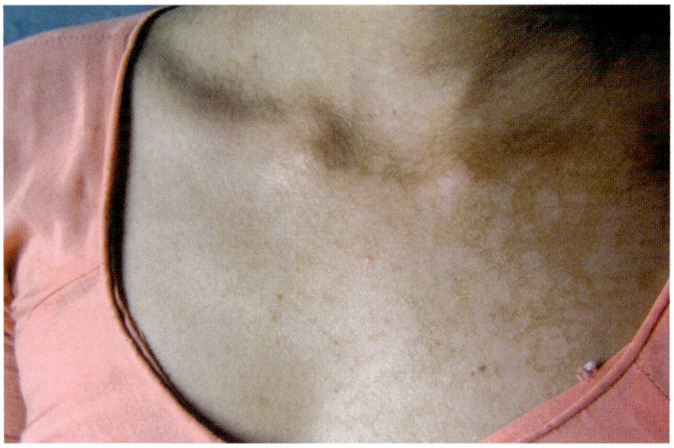

Fig. 3.45: Pityriasis versicolor

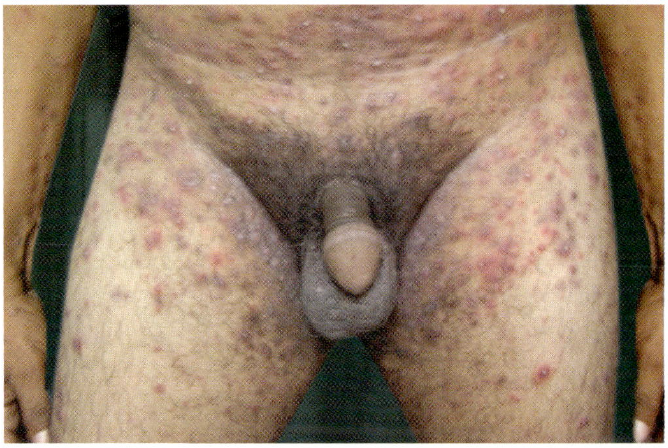

Fig. 3.46: Candidal intertrigo with cutaneous candidiasis—typical vesiculopustules affecting inguinal region and trunk

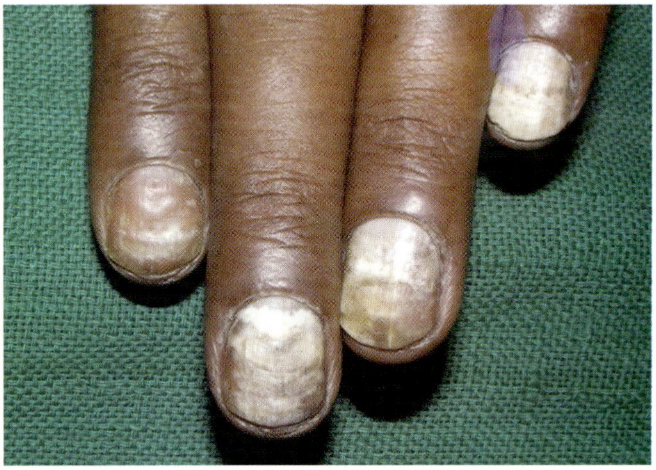

Fig. 3.47: Proximal white superficial onychomycosis

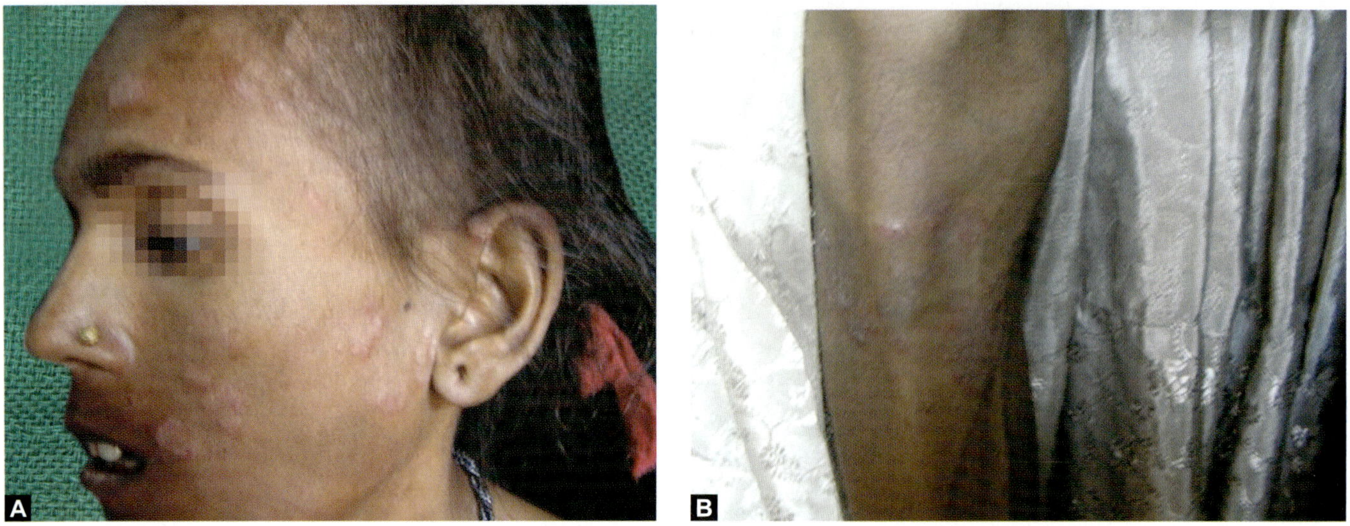

Figs 3.48A and B: (A) Tinea capitis with T. faciei; (B) T. corporis in adult

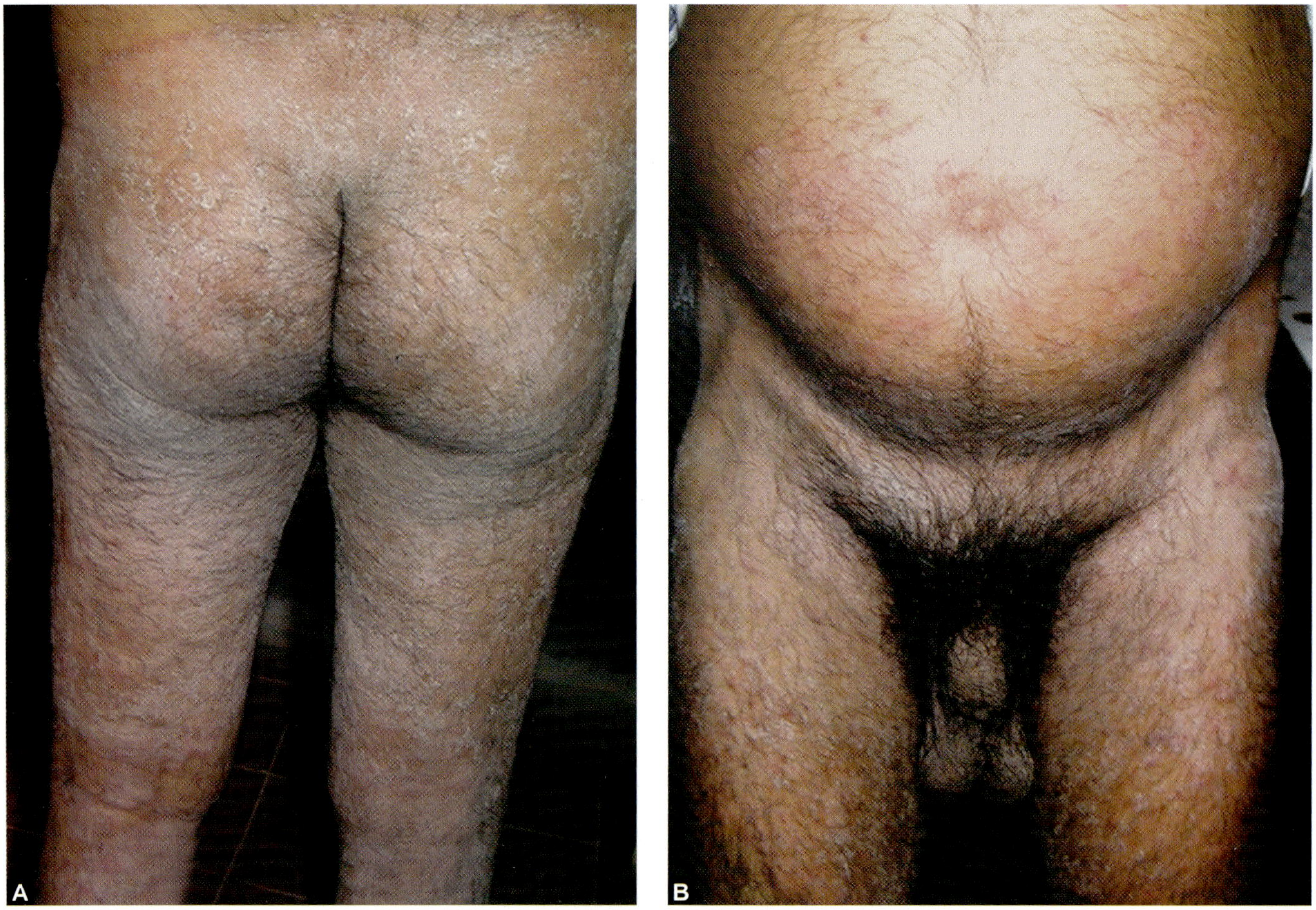

Figs 3.49A and B: Extensive Tinea corporis

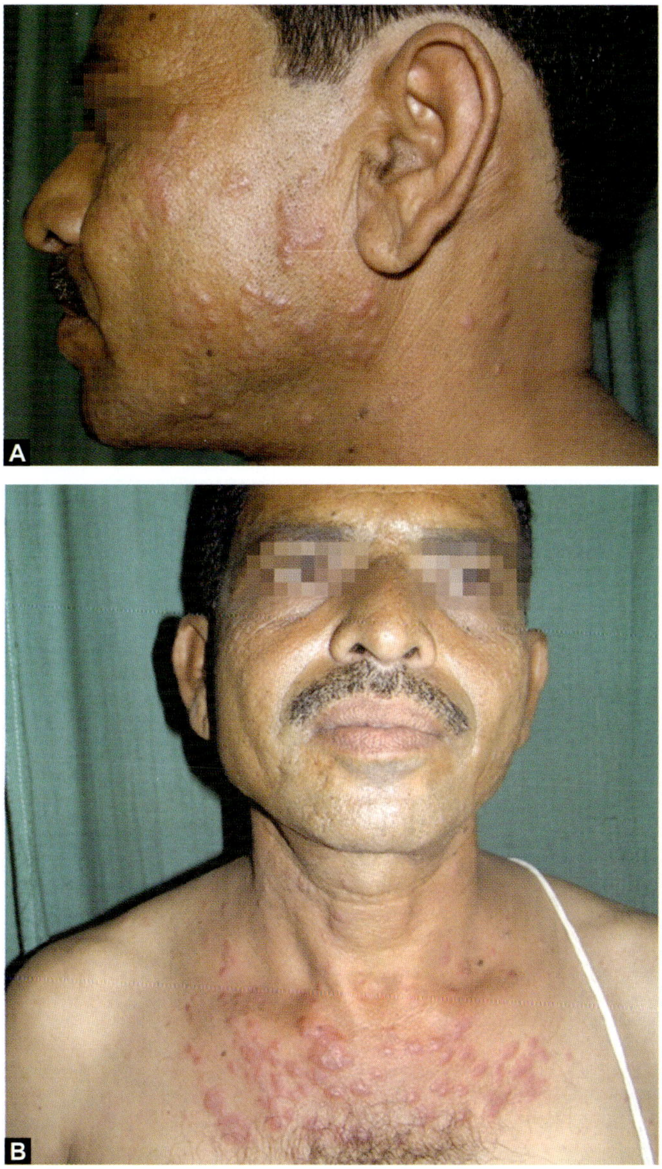

Figs 3.50A and B: (A) Patient with pityrosporum folliculitis presenting with multiple pruritic papular and pustular lesions over the face; (B) Neck of a patient with HIV

as a diffuse erythema (atrophic type) of the oral mucosa involving the palate and tongue or as a non separable plaque or as an angular chelitis. Esophageal candidiasis is an AIDS defining illness.

Pityrosporum ovale causes tinea versicolor (Fig. 3.45), Pityrosporum folliculitis (Fig. 3.50) and seborrheic dermatitis. P. folliculitis is characterized by papular/pustular lesions over face, scalp, trunk and proximal

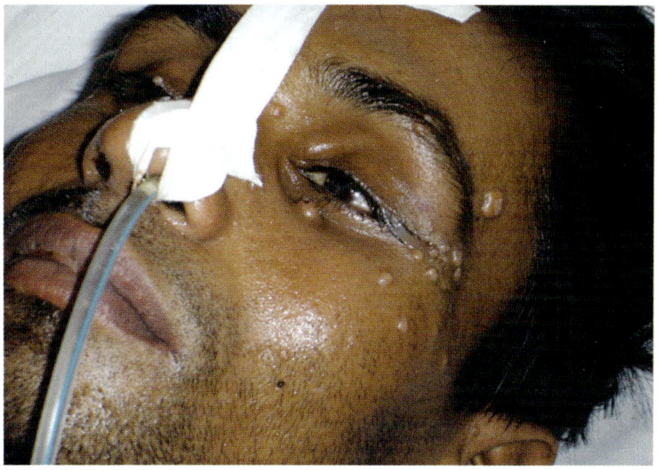

Fig. 3.51: Cutaneous cryptococcosis in a patient of cryptococcal meningitis. Multiple dome shaped umbilicated lesions

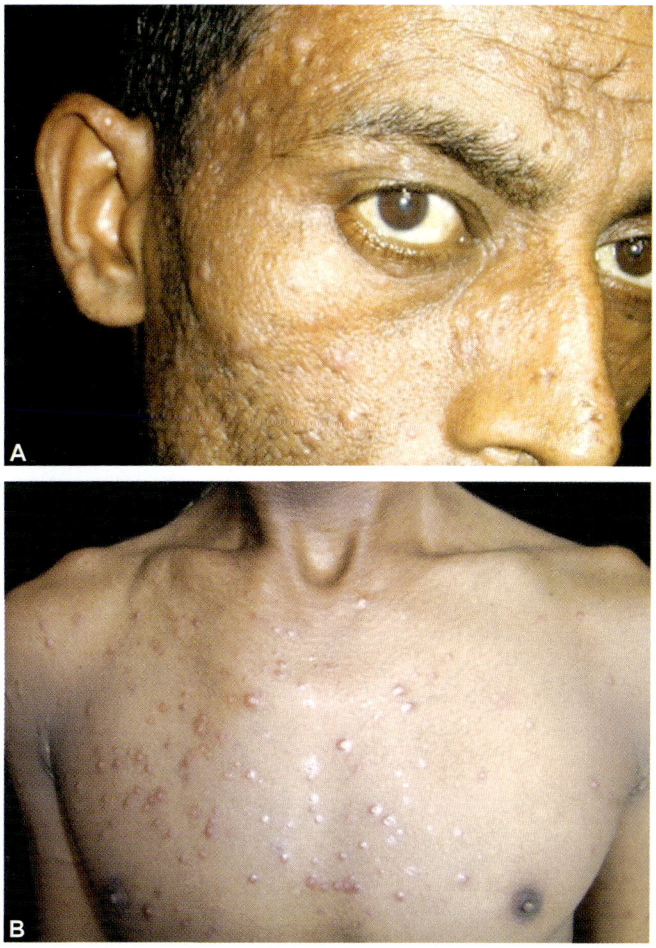

Figs 3.52A and B: Demodex folliculitis presents as a pruritic papular eruption involving the face and neck

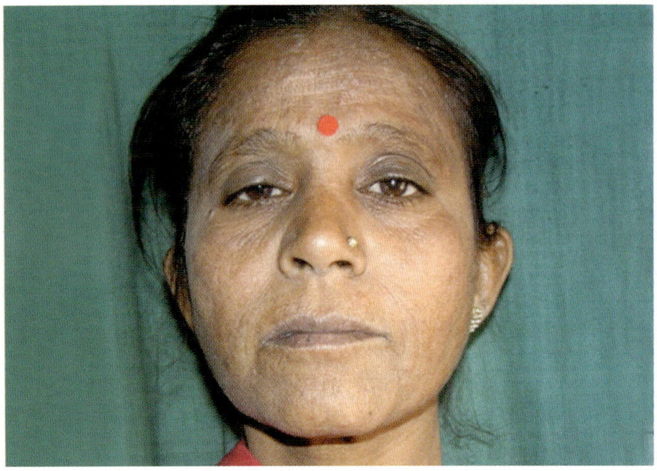

Fig. 3.53: Demodicidosis

arms. It is treated with low potency corticosteroids and topical antifungals. Severe cases are treated by systemic antifungals Ketoconazole, Itraconazole, Terbinafine write dose.

Most common deep fungal infection in HIV/AIDS is cryptococcosis (Fig. 3.51). Cutaneous primary infection is seen in 10–20% cases and it usually follows systemic infection. Intravenous Amphotericin B (0.5–1mg/kg/day) with/without flucytosine dose for 14 days followed by oral fluconazole (400–800 mg/day) for 10 weeks is very much effective. Cryptococcal meningitis is associated with poor prognosis. Lesions present as multiple well-demarcated pink papules that may ulcerate or become pustules at CD4 < 100/microliter. It may present as IRIS in the form of meningitis, pulmonary nodules or lymphadenopathy.

Histoplasmosis, coccidiomycosis, aspergillosis, penicilliosis are the other deep fungal infections that can give rise to cutaneous manifestations in HIV positive patients.

PARASITIC INFESTATIONS

Scabies is common parasitic (Fig. 3.55) infection in HIV positive patients.

Severe and unusual forms of scabies can be seen as papular, atypical or Norwegian (Fig. 3.54) (Crusted) scabies. Atypical scabies is characterized by severe pruritus and papular eruption each topped by a scabetic burrow.

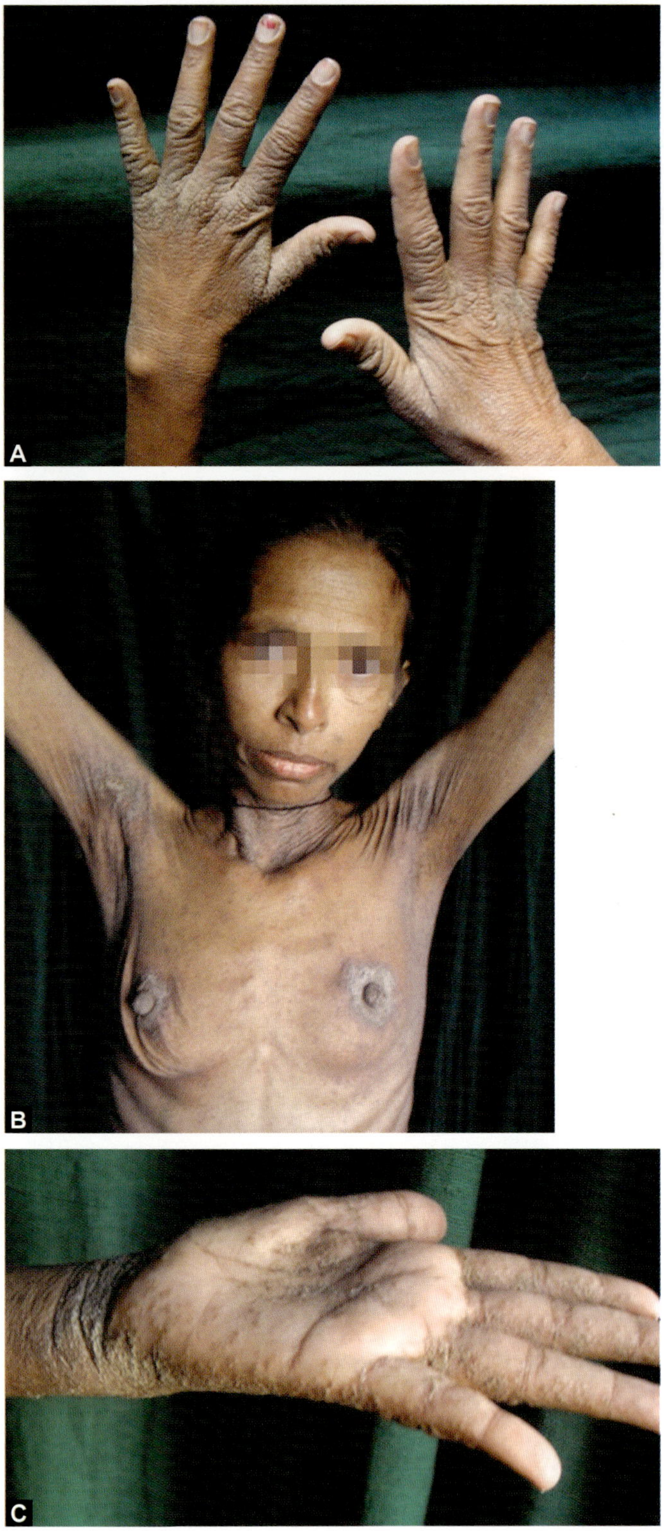

Figs 3.54A to C: Crusted (Norwegian) scabies in PLHA female: (A) Lichenification on dorsum of hands; (B) Involvement of flexures; (C) Involvement of palm i.e. not case in adults

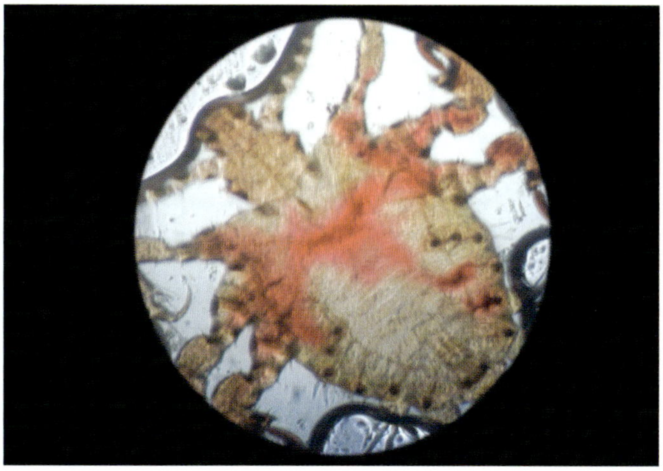

Fig. 3.55: Scabies mite

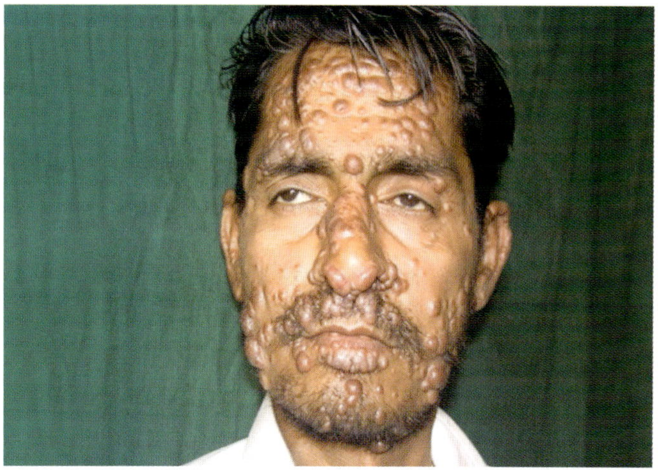

Fig. 3.56: Diffuse cutaneous leishmaniasis

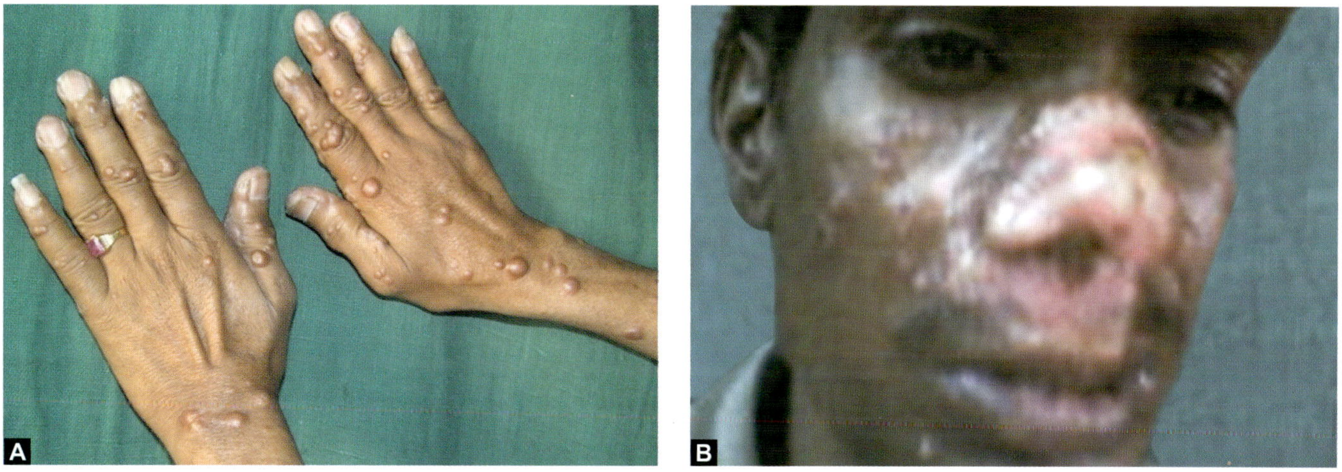

Figs 3.57A and B: Primary cutaneous leishmaniasis

Crusted scabies in severe immunocompromised patients may present as grey white crusted plaques with fissuring and invovlvement of scalp, face, neck, buttocks, nail, etc. Mites as many as a thousand may be recovered from these crusted lesions. Topical treatment is same as in normal course including GBHC, permethrin 5%. Oral Ivermectin is also used. Keratolytics can be used in crusted scabies.

Demodicidosis (demodex folliculitis) (Figs 3.52 and 3.53) is mainly limited to face and neck. Treatment includes lindane 1%, permethrin 1%, sulfur 10%, benzyl benzoate 10%, pilocarpine gel or 5% benzoyl peroxide. Oral drugs include ivermectin (200 μg/kg) and metronidazole.

Leishmaniasis can present with cutaneous (Figs 3.56 and 3.57) or systemic features with a multitude of species as a causative.

4 Sexually Transmitted Infections in HIV/AIDS

Testing and treatment of sexually transmitted infections (STIs) can be an effective tool in preventing the spread of HIV, the virus that causes AIDS. An understanding of the relationship between STIs and HIV infection can help in the development of effective HIV prevention programs for persons with high-risk sexual behaviors.

Individuals who are infected with STIs are about two to five times more likely than uninfected individuals to acquire HIV infection if they are exposed to the virus through sexual contact. In addition, if an HIV-infected individual is also infected with another STI, that person is more likely to transmit HIV through sexual contact than other HIV-infected persons.

There is a substantial biological evidence demonstrating that the presence of other STIs increases the likelihood of both transmitting and acquiring HIV.

INCREASED INFECTIOUSNESS

Sexually transmitted infections (STIs) appear to increase the risk of an HIV-infected person transmitting the virus to his or her sex partners. Studies have shown that HIV-infected individuals who are also infected with other STIs are particularly likely to shed HIV in their genital secretions. For example, men who are infected with both gonorrhea and HIV are more than twice as likely to have HIV in their genital secretions than are those who are infected only with HIV. Moreover, the median concentration of HIV in semen is as much as 10 times higher in men, who are infected with both gonorrhea and HIV, than in men infected only with HIV. The higher the concentration of HIV in semen or genital fluids, the more likely it is that HIV will be transmitted to a sex partner.

INCREASED SUSCEPTIBILITY

STIs appear to increase susceptibility to HIV infection by two mechanisms. Genital ulcers (e.g. syphilis, herpes, or chancroid) result in breaks in the genital tract lining or skin. These breaks create a portal of entry for HIV. Additionally, inflammation resulting from genital ulcers or non-ulcerative STIs (e.g. chlamydia, gonorrhea, and trichomoniasis) increase the concentration of cells in genital secretions that can serve as targets for HIV (e.g. CD4 + cells).

VIRAL STIs

Viral STIs have always been a significant problem amongst the various sexually transmitted infections, as an effective antimicrobial therapy is not available to eradicate the virus completely.

They are a chronic problem and expanding its extent with an increased clinical as well as subclinical episodes. Coincident spread and occurrence of HIV is of particular concern.

In the setting of immunosuppression, especially HIV infection, viral STIs behave in a variable manner and can be to difficult to manage.

Various viral STIs seen are:

1. Herpes genitalis.
2. HPV infection—anogenital warts; condyloma acuminata.
3. Molluscum contagiosum.
4. Viral hepatitis.
5. CMV infection.
6. Epstein Barr virus.
7. HHV 8 infection.

HERPES GENITALIS

This infection, primarily of young adults, can be caused by both HSV 1 or 2. The disease has a high psychosocial impact with a property of recurrences. The severity of clinical presentation and frequency of recurrences are influenced both by host as well as viral factors;

- Gender
- Immune status
- Viral type
- Prior immunity to autologus or heterologus virus.

Common presentations of herpes genitalis(HP) are:

- Vesicular lesions associated with pain and tenderness (Fig. 4.1)
- Genital ulcers
- Perianal and anal ulcers
- Fissuring of vulva, perianal region
- Cervicitis/proctitis
- Discharge from urethra, vagina, rectum
- Painless ulcers at time
- Asymptomatic lesions sometimes.

Atypical presentation of HP seen in HIV:

- Atypical site-buttocks, lower back, medial aspect of thigh (Fig. 4.2)
- Progressive ulcers
- Deep ulceration (Fig. 4.5)
- Hemorrhagic ulcers
- Hyperkeratotic lesions(like condyloma lata)
- Increased duration and severity of disease
- Pseudotumor of tongue
- Esophagitis, hepatitis, pneumonitis, disseminated infection associated with viremia
- Continuous and prolonged shedding
- Increased recurrences.

HIV 1 infected persons are more commonly infected with HSV 1 type. Various types and variations of clinical manifestations have already been mentioned. However, a new syndrome, immune reconstitution inflammatory syndrome (IRIS) is seen emerging with the introduction of HAART (Highly active antiretroviral therapy). IRIS is seen mainly with advanced immunosuppression (CD4 count < 200/mm^3).

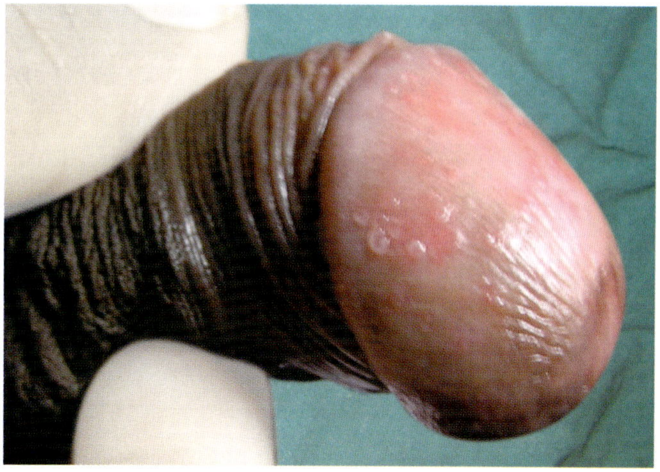

Fig. 4.1: Vesicular lesions of herpes progenitalis with erythema over glans

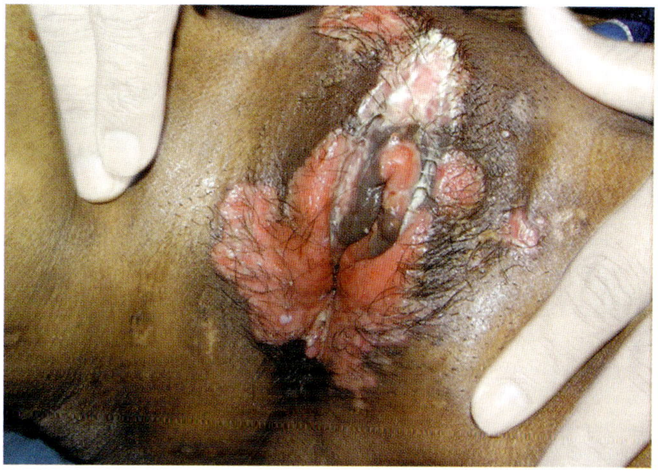

Fig. 4.2: Necrotic herpes genitalis in a female patient

Management

HIV-infected patients are more prone to develop recurrence of HSV when compared to normal population. Suppressive therapy with acyclovir, valacyclovir or famciclovir decreases the frequency and severity of HSV 2 recurrences and asymptomatic HSV 2 reactivation. These antiviral drugs are safe and effective in persons with HIV 1 infection. They additionally benefit by decreasing HIV 1 levels in persons coinfected with HIV 1 and HSV 2.

Episodic Treatment

- Acyclovir 400 mg tid orally for 5–10 days (Figs 4.3 and 4.4)
- Famciclovir 500 mg bid orally for 5–10 days
- Valacyclovir 1.0 g bid orally for 5–10 days.

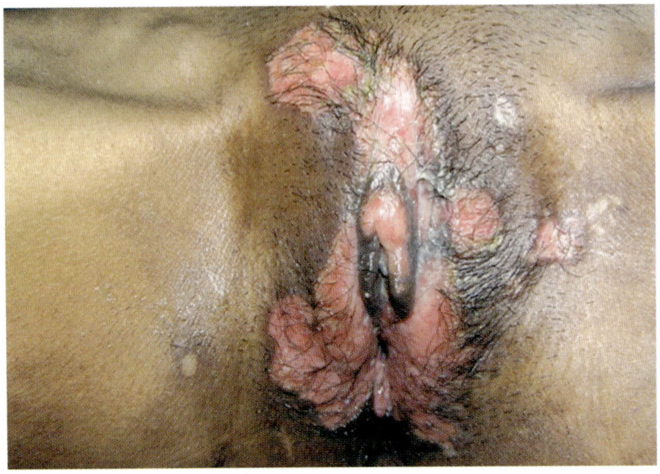

Fig. 4.3: Follow-up of the patient in Figure 4.2 after 6 days of acyclovir therapy

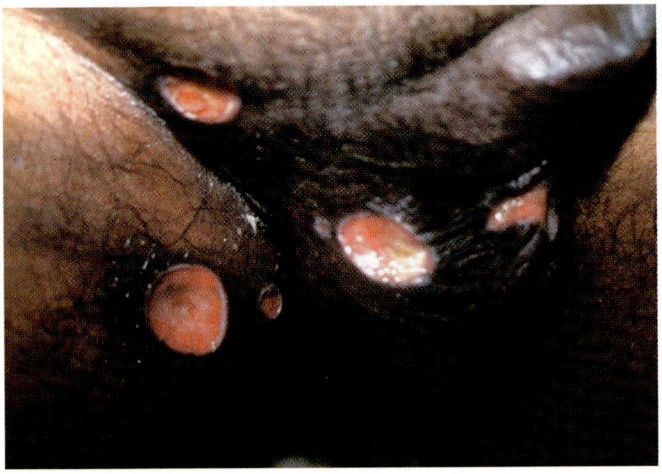

Fig. 4.5: Deep necrotic herpetic ulcers present on the scrotum and groin sparing penis

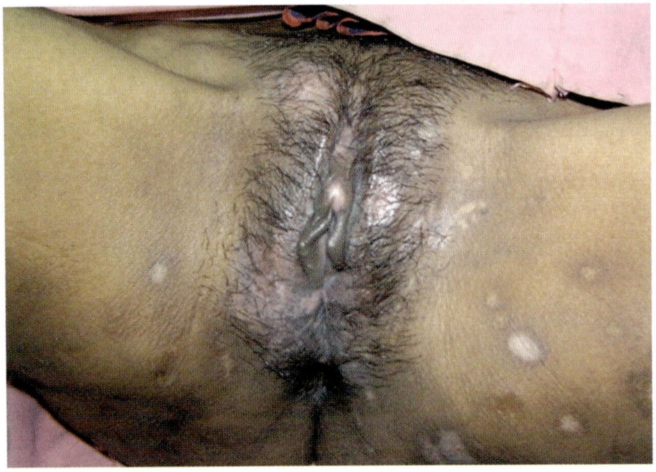

Fig. 4.4: Follow-up of the same patient after a 10 days course of acyclovir

Suppressive Therapy

- Acyclovir 400–800 mg bid/tid
- Famciclovir 500 mg orally bid
- Valacyclovir 500 mg orally bid to be continued from 6 months upto 2 years.

Resistance is suspected if lesions persist in a patient receiving antiviral treatment.

Acyclovir Resistant HSV

- Foscarent 40 mg/kg body weight IV 8 hourly until clinical resolution
- Topical cidofovir gel 1% for 5 days might be effective.

HUMAN PAPILLOMA VIRUS INFECTION ANOGENITAL WARTS; CONDYLOMA ACUMINATA

They are one of the mot common STIs, the infecton is subclinical initially and no modality of treatment eliminates the virus. HPV targets epithelial cells and the replication of virus depends on presence of differentiating squamous epithelium. Clinical and histopathological appearance is seen at 1–8 months after initial exposure. Persistence may be attributed to decreased local immunological response.

Increase in the cell mediated immunity (CMI) is thought to be effective in regression, control of reactivation, preventing recurrence and elimination of warts. Thus patients with decreased CMI, including HIV patients have an increased incidence of warts.

Clinical presentation remains the same in HIV-infected and non HIV-infected persons. However, the lesions can be bigger, florid and resistant to treatment in HIV-infected individuals (Figs 4.6 to 4.9, 4.13, 4.47).

In HIV-infected persons, warts can present in a florid manner at even extragenital sites (Fig. 4.10). In-fact, the appearance of florid warts can be a clue to investigate and detect a new HIV positive case.

HPV is largely known to be a predisposing agent in the causation of CIN (cervical intraepithelial neoplasia), VIN (vulval intraepithelial neoplasia). High anal carcinoma, which can be due to prior HPV infection, is

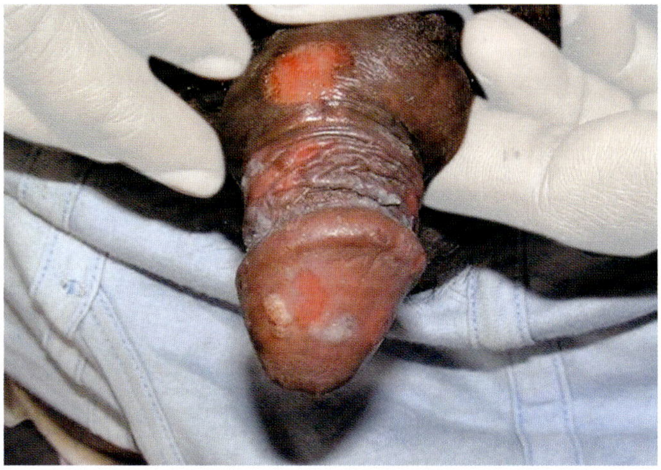

Fig. 4.6: Mixed STI with lesions of herpes progenitalis and genital warts. This is quite common in reactive patients

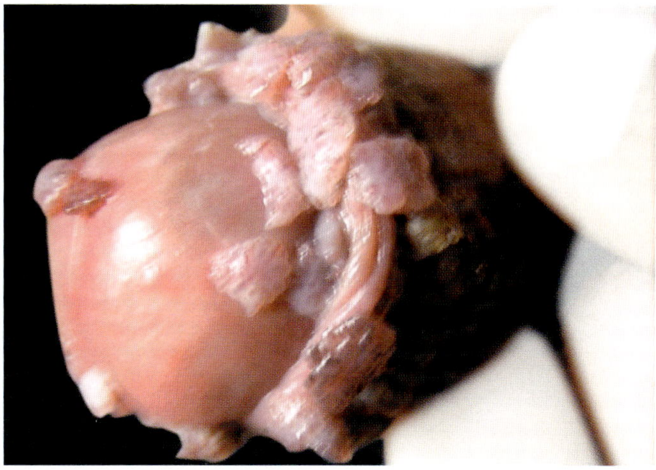

Fig. 4.8: Multiple genital warts present over glans, undersurface of prepuce and preputial skin

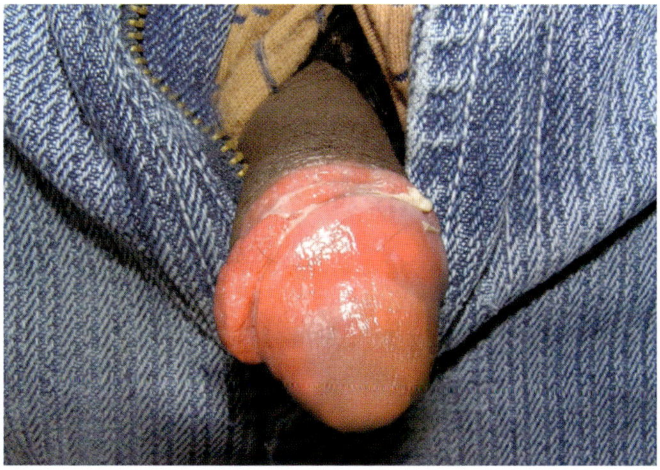

Fig. 4.7: Vascular type of condyloma acuminata at coronal sulcus in a HIV positive patient

an AIDS defining illness. However, early HPV infection can be detected by a simple procedure with aceto-whitening staining and PAP smear.

Treatment options are same as in non HIV-infected persons, which include:

- Podophyllotoxin-20%
- Imiquimod
- Cold steel surgery
- Scissors excision
- Electrosurgery
- Laser excision

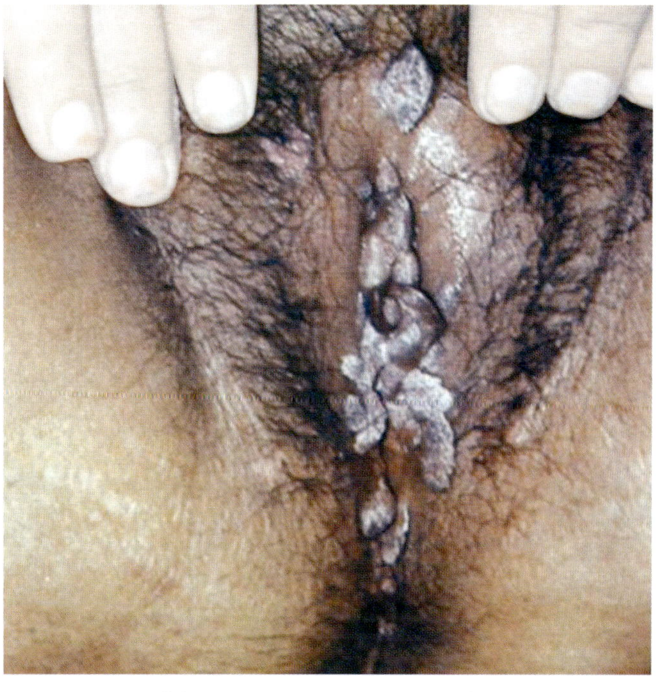

Fig. 4.9: Condyloma acuminata—verrucous lesions over labia majora, minora and fourchette

- Cryotherapy (Fig. 4.11)
- Trichloracetic acid.

Recently HPV vaccine has been introduced as a preventive vaccine for HPV infection, keeping in thought the role of this virus in causation of cervical

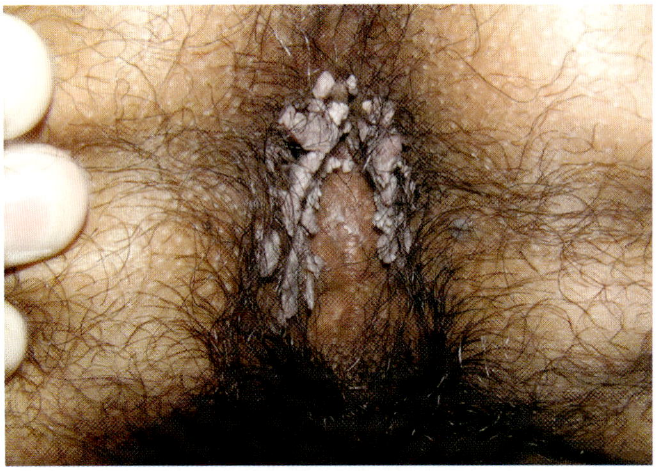

Fig. 4.10: Perianal warts

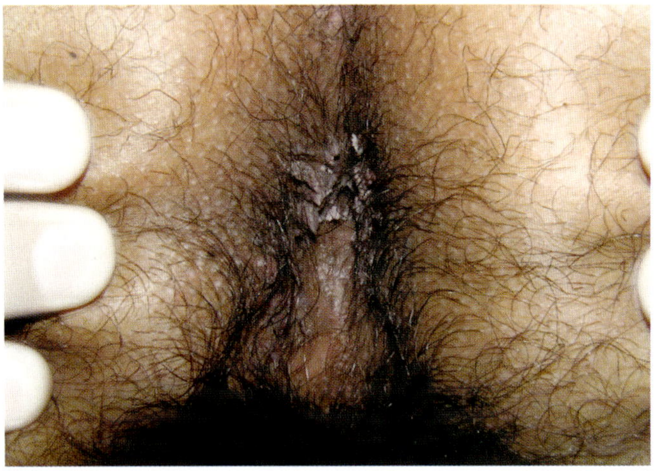

Fig. 4.11: Follow-up of the patient in Figure 4.9 after 3 weeks of cryotherapy

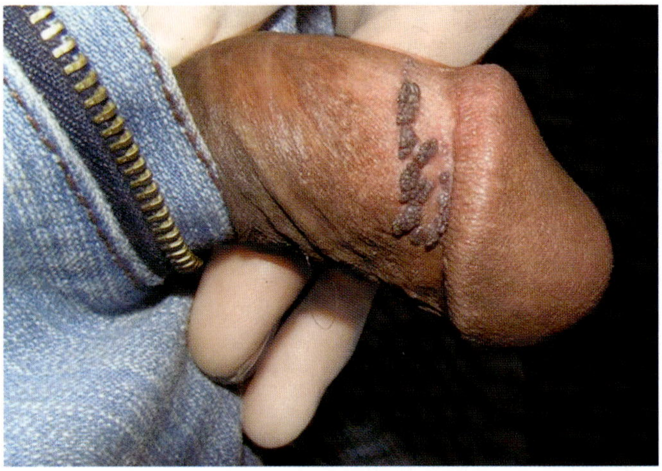

Fig. 4.13: Bowenoid papulosis

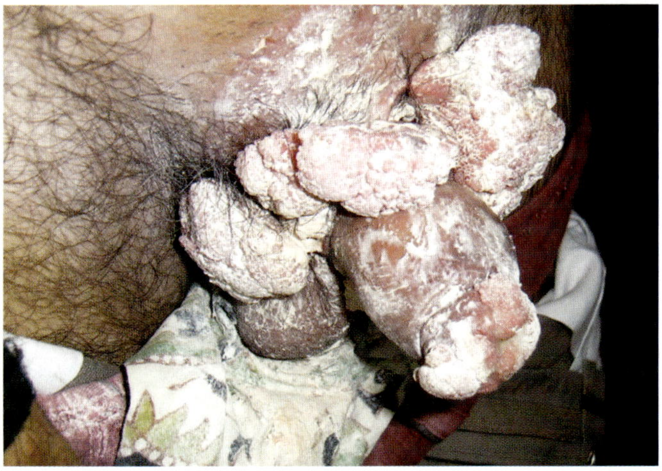

Fig. 4.12: Buschke-Lowenstein tumor

cancer—the most common carcinoma in females in India. Vaccine is against the 6, 11, 16, 18 HPV subtypes.

Patient counseling and regular screening to rule out cervical carcinoma or *in situ* carcinoma cervix has to be done in patients with HPV infection.

Buschke-Lowenstein Tumor : is a squamous cell tumor arising out of pre-existing condyloma Acuminata (HPV type 6, 11, 16, 18) (Fig. 4.12).

MOLLUSCUM CONTAGIOSUM

Molluscum contagiosum (MC) is a benign papular condition and a commonly seen sexually transmitted infection in young adults. However , the virus cannot be grown in cell culture, may be because of its need of highly differentiated keratinocytes.

Although out of the four subtypes, MC 1, 2, 3 and 4, MC 1 is more common epidemiologically, in HIV infected persons, MC 2 subtype is more commonly seen. Attendence for MC virus infection is more amongst HIV/AIDS patients than non infected patients.

Clinical presentation (Figs 4.14 and 4.15) is almost similar in both HIV infected and non infected persons but there many be increase in number and size of lesions (Fig. 4.16). MC lesions may also commonly become giant (10–15 mm) and ulcerated in HIV-infected

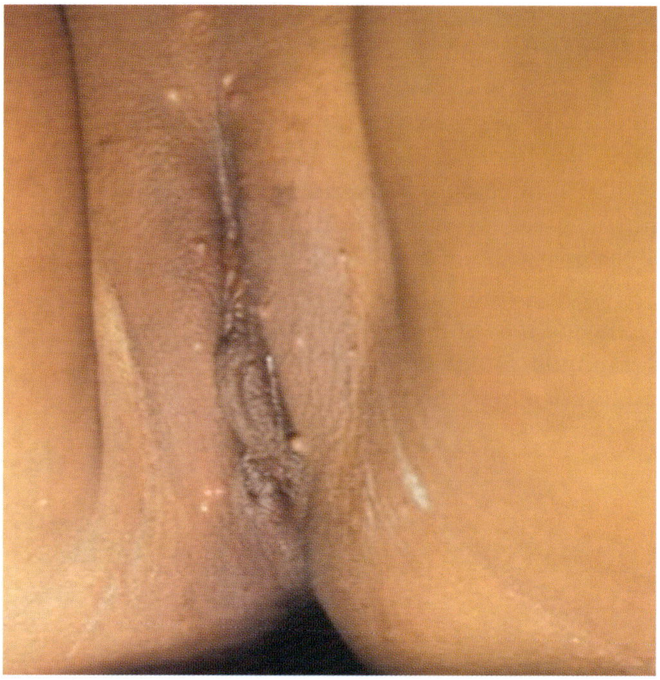

Fig. 4.14: Molluscum contagiosum—white pearly lesions present over vulva and labia majora

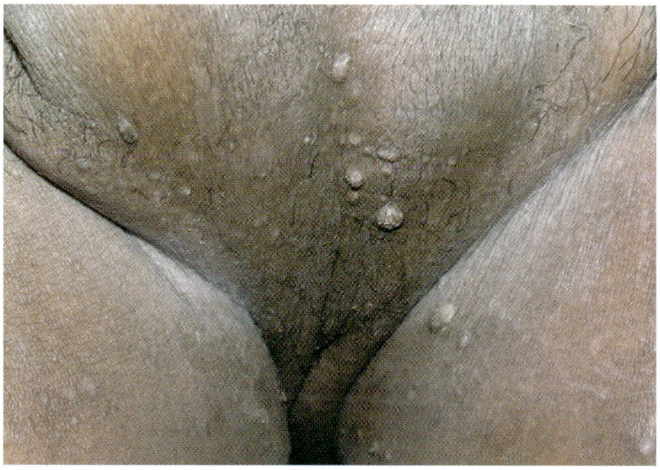

Fig. 4.15: Molluscum contagiosum over pubic, suprapubic region and thigh of a reactive female patient

persons. They should be differentiated from systemic fungal infections like cryptococcosis, histoplasmosis, penicilliosis in HIV seropositive patients, especially on face. The occurrence of these lesions can be seen as a presentation of IRIS.

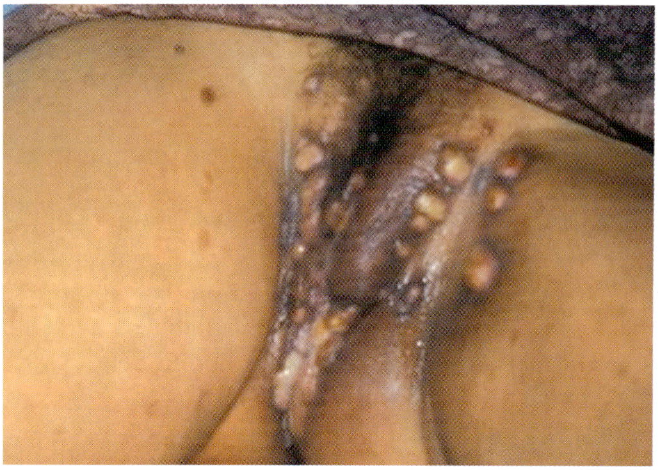

Fig. 4.16: Giant molluscum present in a female patient with serum HIV positive. Post-inflammatory hyperpigmentation present at the site of prior cryotherapy

Normally, the lesions are self-limiting and may get cleared spontaneously, with treatment modalities include curettage, cauterization, cryotherapy with liquid N2, phenol, KOH (10%), imiquimod, etc. But in HIV infected patients, the lesions are nonresponsive and resistant. They may clear up with ongoing anti retroviral therapy and improvement in CMI of the patient.

OTHER VIRAL STIs

Viral Hepatitis A, B, C, cytomegalo virus infection and HHV 8 infection do not commonly present with mucocutaneous manifestations, but systemic involvement. However, if present, CMV may cause persistent ulcers in genital and perianal area.

BACTERIAL STIs

Chancroid

It is an acute, autoinoculable and usually localized genital ulcer disease(GUD), caused by *Haemophilus ducreyi*.

Chancroid, also termed 'ulcus molle,' is a disease primarily of sexually promiscuous individual\s and males are more commonly affected than females.

Both humoral and cell mediated immunity (CMI) are supposed to be involved as a protective immunity in chancroid. Th1 cells are the predominant CMI mediators with a paucity of B lymphocytes lineage.

Generally, high IgG titre and decreased lymphocyte response to *Haemophilus ducreyi* are found in HIV-infected patients as compared to non infected patients.

Usual clinical presentation is of a soft tender papule with erythematous halo which evolves into a pustule, erosion and ulcer within 24–48 hours. Ulcer may be single or multiple (might be a result of autoinoculation). Ulcer, in chancroid (Fig. 4.19), is non indurated, tender and covered with yellowish exudates, which may bleed on manipulation, Phimosis/paraphimosis can be seen (Figs 4.18 and 4.20). Tender inguinal lymphadenitis (usually unilateral) and unilocular abcess (bubo) can be seen (Fig. 4.21).

In HIV-infected person chancroid may present in a more severe and altered form:

- Extensive necrotizing lesion or phagedenic chancroid (Figs 4.17 and 4.19)
- Maggot infestation
- Multiple/multilocular buboes (Fig. 4.20)
- Slow healing

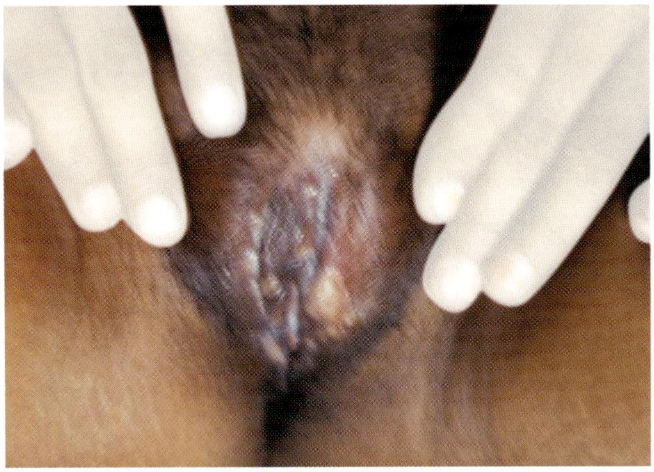

Fig. 4.17: Chancroid-ulcer with reactionary edema

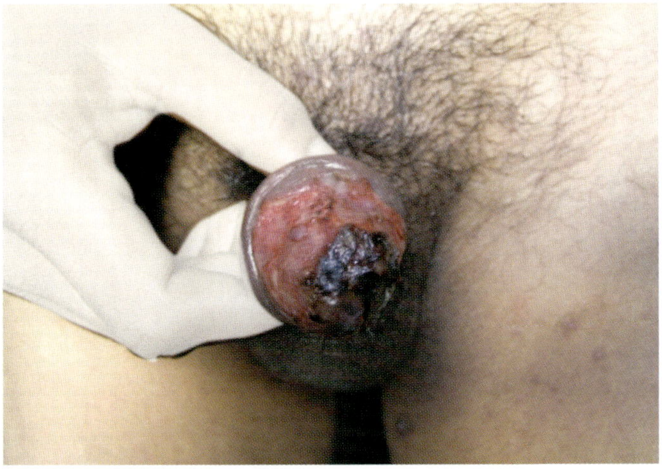

Fig. 4.19: Phagedenic chancroid

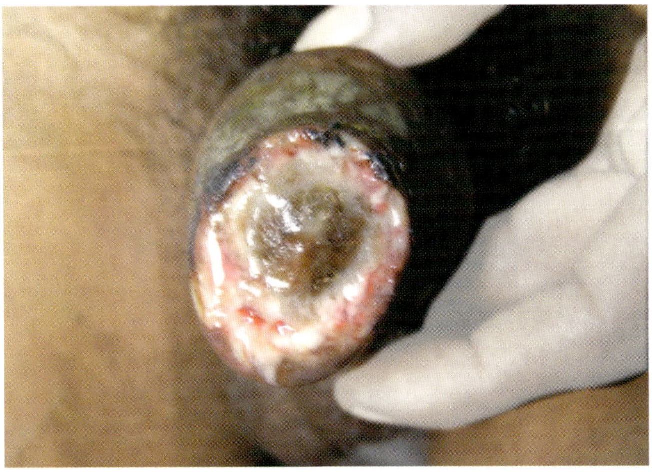

Fig. 4.18: Phimosis with subpreputial discharge—there was tender lymphadenopathy and history of single ulcer over glans

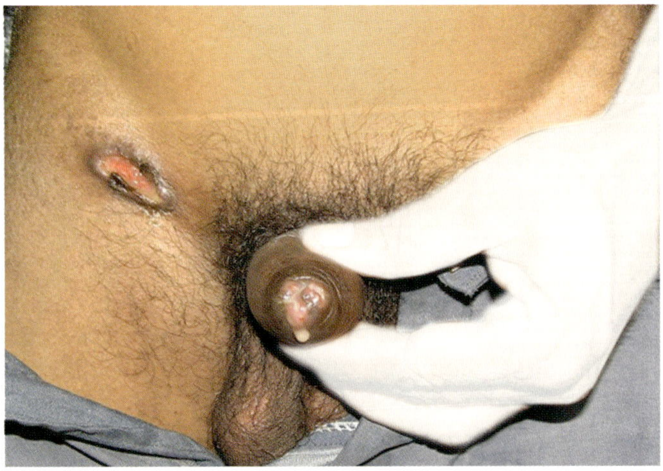

Fig. 4.20: Phimosis with subpreputial discharge causing soiling of pants with ruptured bubo suggestive of chancroid

- Longer duration of treatment
- Treatment failure.

Sometimes some genital ulcers may present with lesions similar to chancroid ulcer, but they are not caused by the organism, *Haemphilus ducreyi*, they are termed chancroidal ulcers.

Treatment regimens are no different in HIV infected or non infected persons. Commonly used drugs are as per the following regimen:

- Erythromycin stearate/base—500 mg qid for 7 days
- Erythromycin ethyl succinate—800 mg qid for 7 days
- Ciprofloxacin—500 mg bid for 3-5 days
- Ceftriaxone—250 mg im stat
- Azithromycin—1 g stat dose
- Doxycycline—100 mg bid for 7 days trimethoprin (80 mg) + sulfamethoxazole (400 mg 2 tab bid for 14 days).

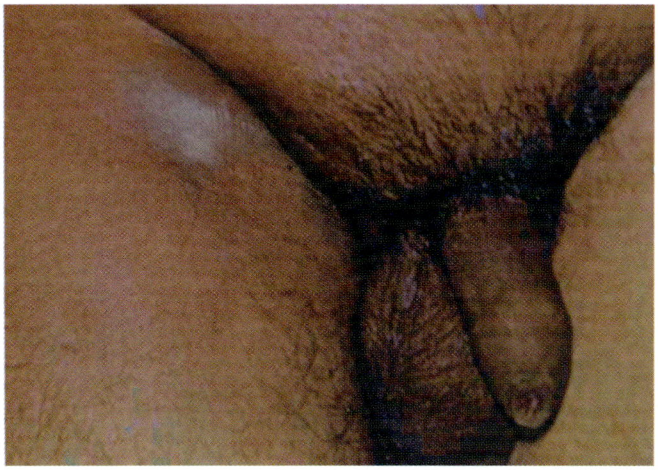

Fig. 4.21: Typical sign of groove of greenblatt with enlarged inguinal lymph nodes separated by Poupart's ligament

LYMPHOGRANULOMA VENERUM

It is a chronic systemic disease that begins at the site of inoculation, usually genitalia, and advances via lymphatics. Causative organism of lymphogranuloma venerum (LGV) is chlamydia trachomatis L1, L2, L3 types.

The disease is characterized by development of suppurative regional lymphadenitis, which is usually preceded by a small, fleeting, many atimes unnoticed, primary lesion. Most common type of primary lesion is a herpetiform, superficial, painless, evanescent lesion, which does not leave a scar on healing.

There is enlargement of femoral and inguinal lymph nodes, which are separated by inguinal ligament (Sign of Greenblatt) (Fig. 4.21).

However, localization of the disease is predominantly inguinal in males and genitoanorectal in females, due to the, different lymphatic drainage of the genitalia in both the sexes (Figs 4.22 and 4.23).

Concomitant occurrence of LGV with HIV infection is not seen very commonly. However, occurrence of Perinaud's syndrome (Oculoglandular syndrome) has been reported.

Treatment of LGV in HIV-infected patients does not differ from those of uninfected patients. However, prolonged therapy may be required and resolution may be delayed.

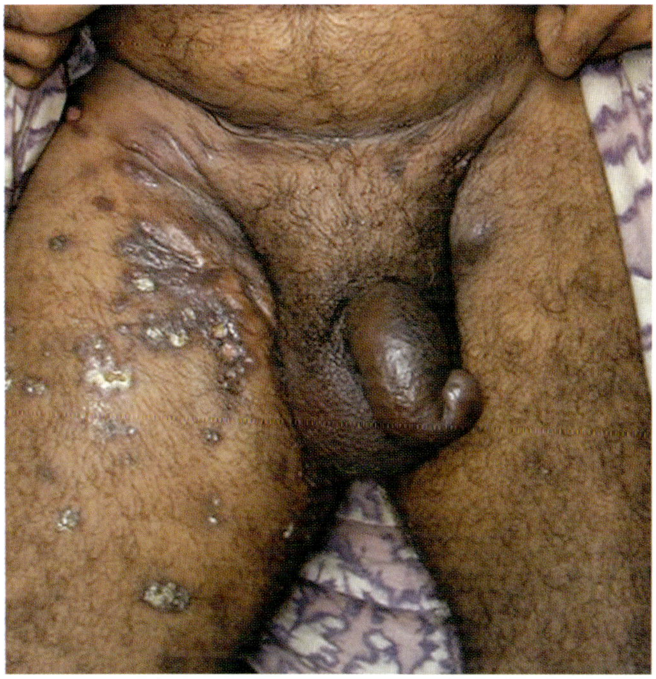

Fig. 4.22: Saxophone penis—a complication of LGV. Note the difference in limb girth of the patient and the scars

Various regimens, which can be used are:

- Doxycycline—100 mg bid for 21 days
- Erythromycin ethyl succinate—800 mg qid for 21 days.

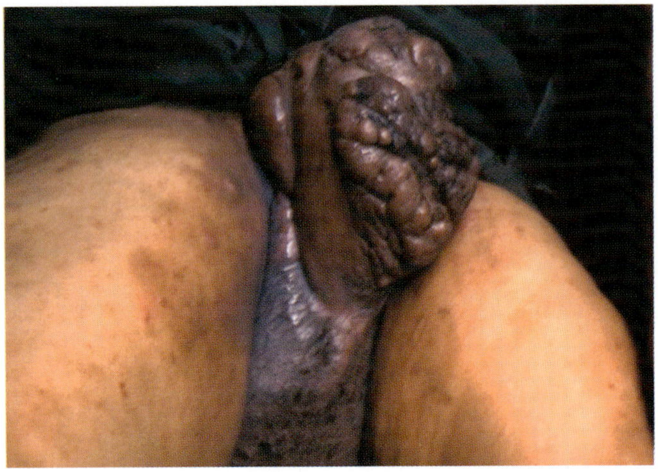

Fig. 4.23: Esthiomene—a late complication of LGV

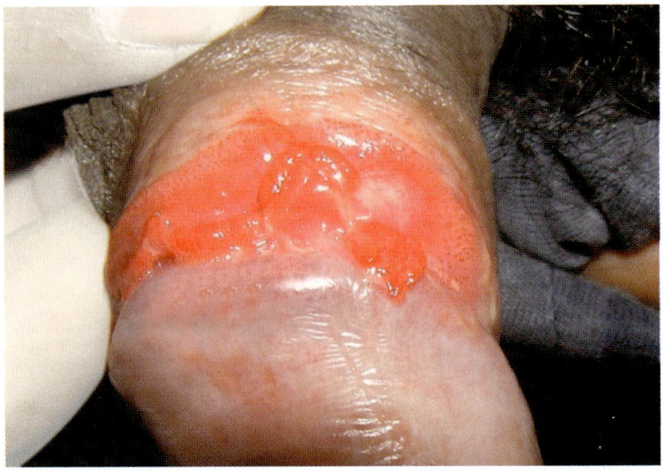

Fig. 4.25 Beefy red ulcer of granuloma inguinale present over coronal sulcus spreading to undersurface of prepuce. Ulcer was non tender and bleed on touch on examination

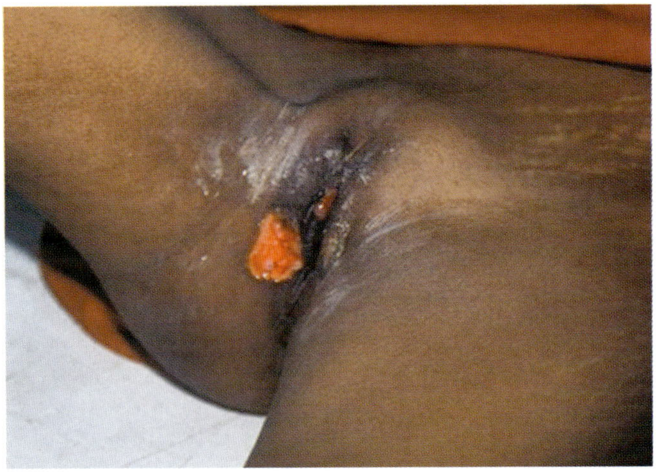

Fig. 4.24: Typically beefy red, granulomatous ulcer of donovanosis present over labia majora in a female patient

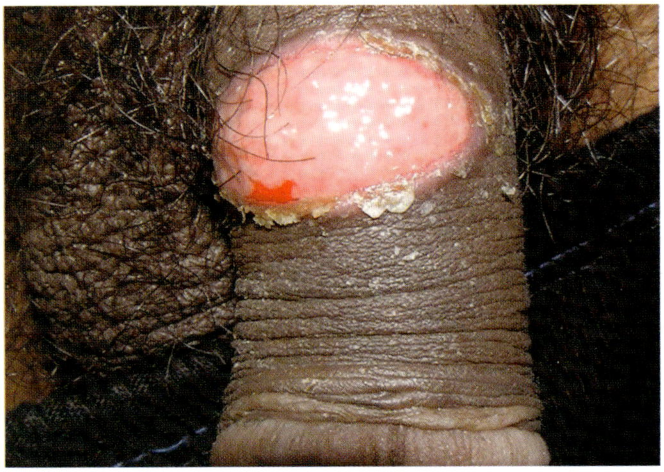

Fig. 4.26: Granuloma inguinale ulcer over shaft of penis; bleeding occurred on lower border after gentle palpation

DONOVANOSIS

This disease is also called as granuloma inguinale (GI). It is a chronic, indolent , sexually transmitted , granulomatous ulceration of genito-inguinal region (Fig. 4.24). Causative organism for GI is *Calymmatobacterium granulomatis* or *Klebsiella granulomatis*.

The basic importance of the disease lies in its one of the important cofactor in facilitating the transmission of HIV infection.

The disease has an affinity for stratified epithelium of cutaneous and mucocutaneous surfaces of the genital, anal and oral region. Initial lesion is a small painless papule or nodule, which may later become swollen and eroded to form sharply circumscribed non-indurated ulcer having a granulomatous base and red beefy everted margins (Figs 2.25 and 4.26). Pain and lymphadenopathy are seen only if secondary infection ensues. Sometimes, early lesion may be a subcutaneous swelling that gradually softens and results in a small abscess (Pseudobubo) with no true lymphadenitis. There are various morphological variants of the disease.

The GUD are important facilitator for transmission of HIV, and this risk is far greater with donovanosis. Rate of HIV seropositivity increases with the duration of the disease. In donovanosis associated with HIV infection, treatment schedules need to be altered because of gross immune suppression. The major variation in the presence of HIV infection is seen in the meantime of healing and tissue destruction associated with ulcers and not the clinical presentation of the lesion or disease itself. However, extragenital dissemination of the disease has been reported in association with HIV infection.

Treatment options are the same in patients with concurrent HIV infection and those who are not. High therapeutic failure rates to the first line antibiotics may be observed.

Commonly used drugs are:
- Doxycycline—100 mg bid for 14 days
- Tetracycline hydrochloride—500 mg qid for 14 days
- Erythromycin stearate or base—500 mg qid for 14 days
- Trimethoprim-sulfamethoaxzole (160-800 mg) bid for 14 days or till lesions have completely healed.

SYPHILIS

Syphilis is a chronic systemic disease caused by *Treponema pallidum*. Syphilis simulates every other disease.

Concurrernt infection of HIV in a patient affects the epidemiology, clinical presentations and even treatment of syphilis.

Clinical features of the disease, as observed in a patient who is also infected with HIV, show few atypical features apart from typical presentations.

Primary Lesions

- Painless ulcer becomes painful due to superadded infection (Fig. 4.27)
- Giant chancre (Fig. 4.28).

Secondary Lesions (Figs 4.29 to 4.40)

Lues maligna: Nodulo ulcerative lesions with features of vasculitis along with fever,malaise, headache (Fig. 4.41).

Course of the Disease

- Shorter latent period
- Rapid progression to tertiary disease (Figs 4.42 and 4.43), especially meningovascular syphilis.

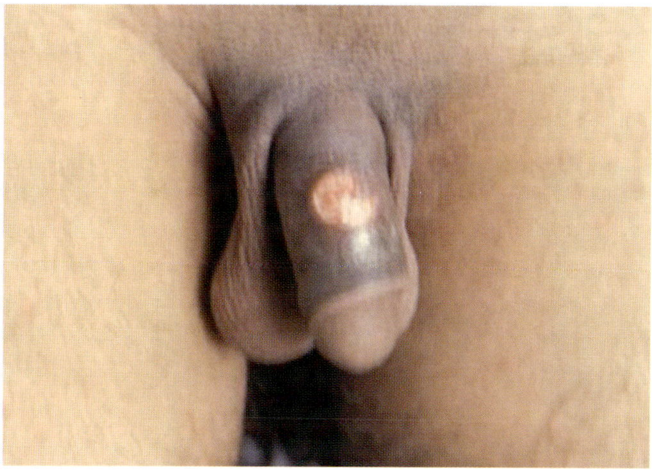

Fig. 4.27 Single ulcer of primary syphilis present at coronal sulcus. The ulcer was asymptomatic, indurated on palpation

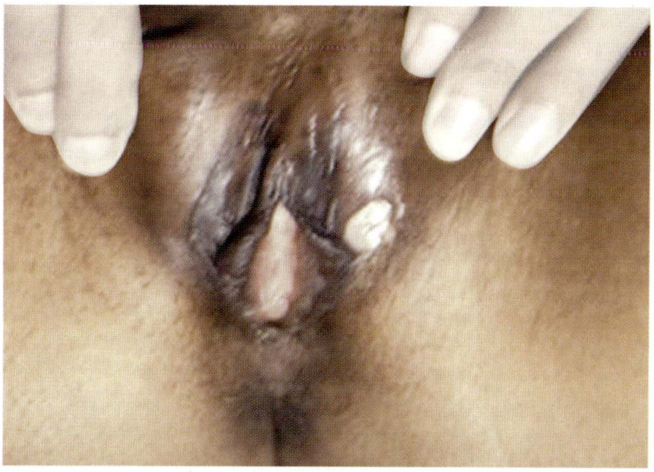

Fig. 4.28: Primary chancre of syphilis

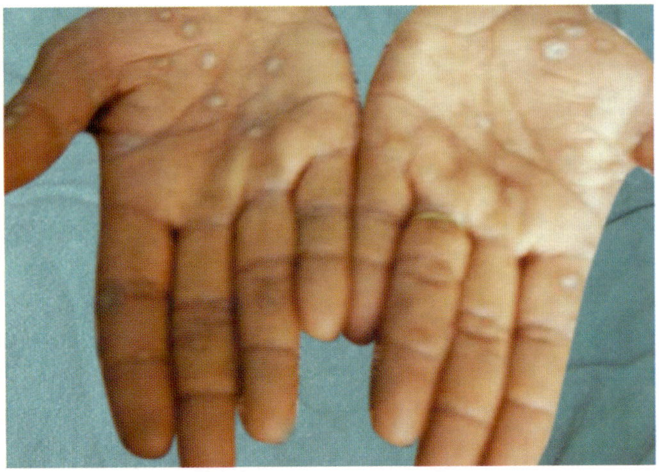

Fig. 4.29: Palmar syphilides

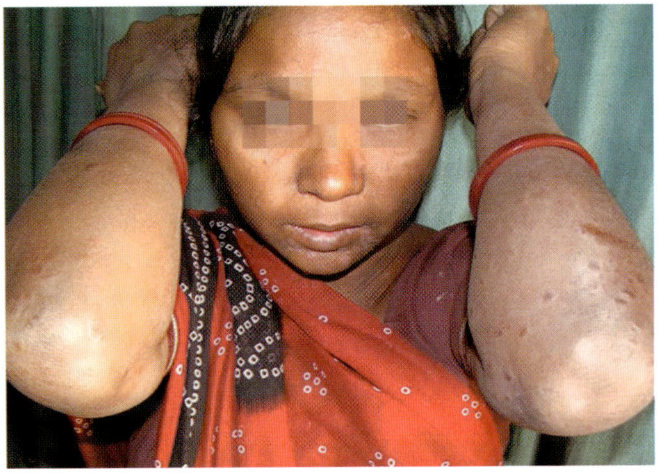

Fig. 4.30: Rash of secondary syphilis in a female with serum HIV positive

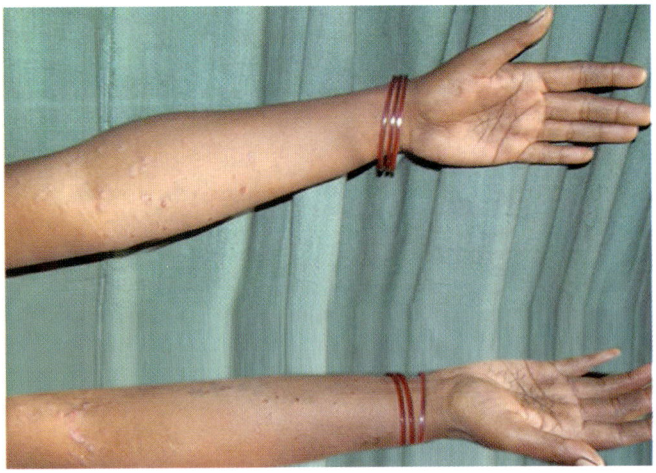

Fig. 4.31: Photograph of the same female in Figure 4.30

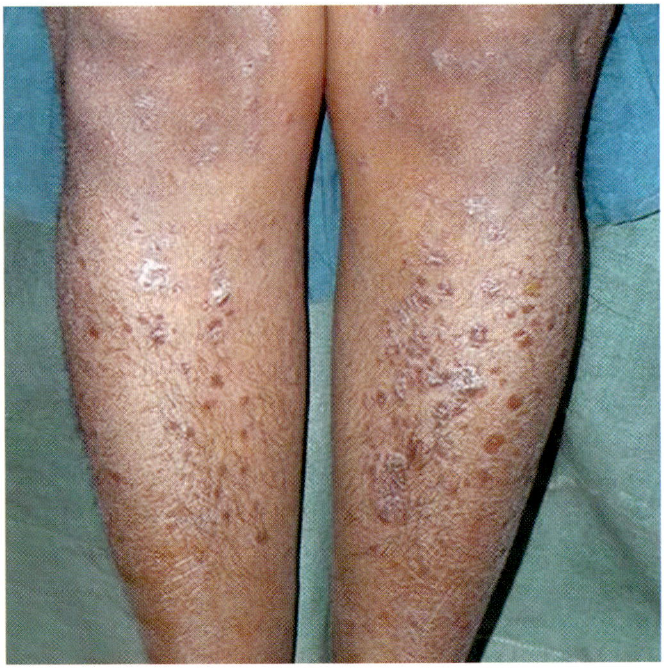

Fig.4.32: Photograph showing shin of the same female in the Figure 4.30 with rash of secondary syphilis

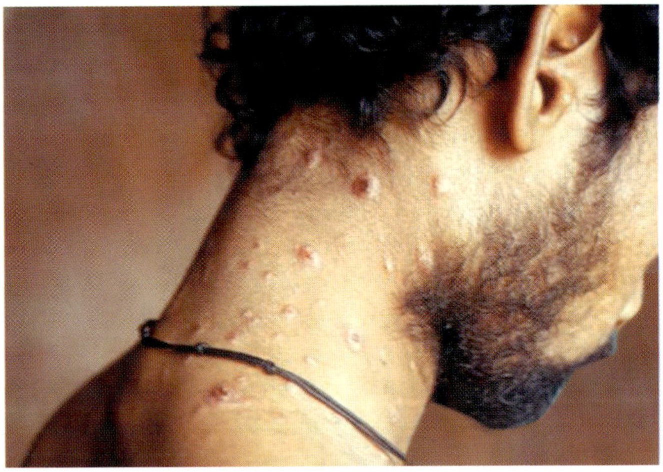

Fig. 4.33: Nodular lesions in secondary syphilis

There are some serological variations seen in syphilis and HIV coinfection. There is limited or absent antibody response to syphilis. The reagin and treponemal antibody testing in serum or CSF can be repeatedly negative. As a result, confirmatory diagnosis can be made only with dark field microscopy, biopsy of

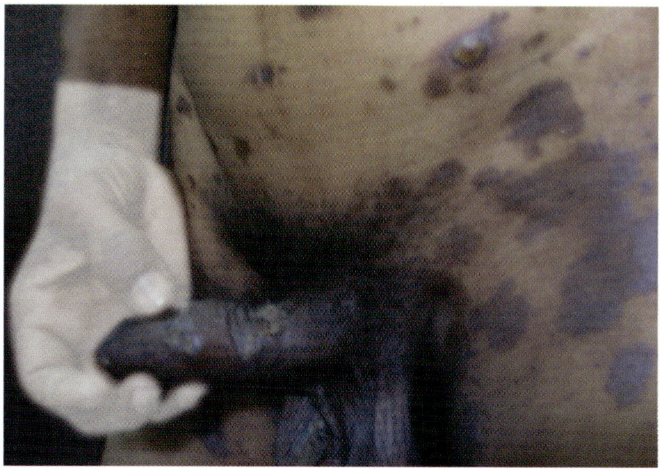

Fig. 4. 34: Psoriasiform rash in secondary syphilis affecting the penis also. The patient was retrogradely detected to be HIV positive

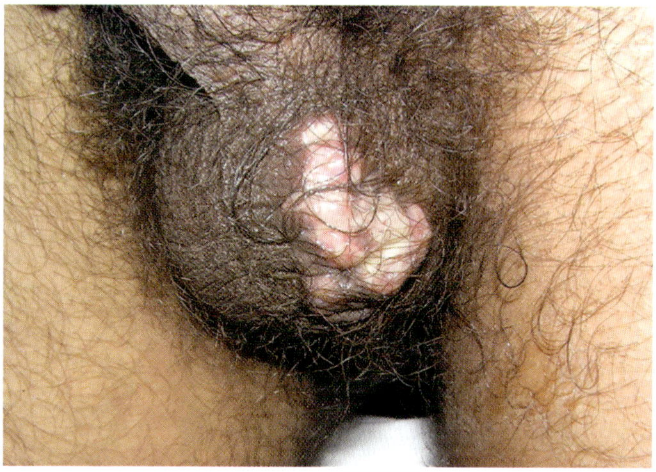

Fig. 4.36: Condyloma lata

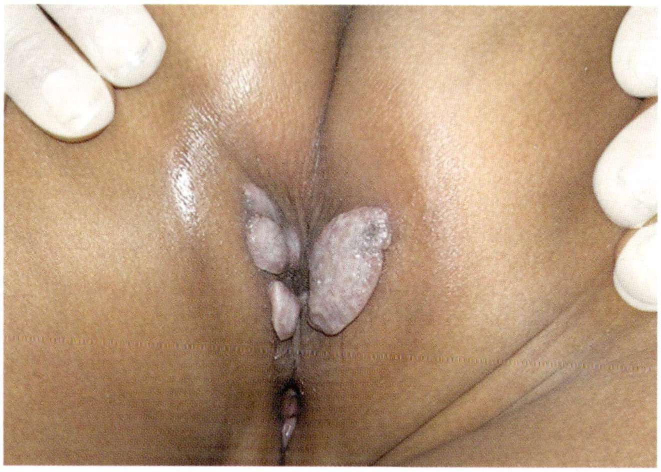

Fig. 4.35: Condyloma lata in perianal region—secondary syphilis

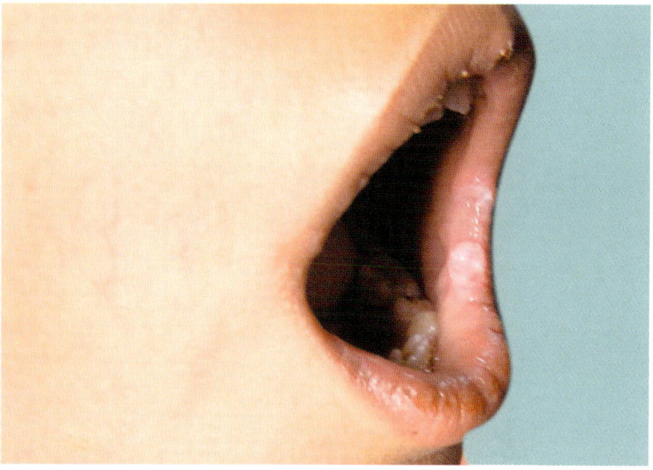

Fig. 4.37: Split papules—another mucosal lesion in secondary syphilis

the lesion or direct fluorescein antibody staining of the material from the lesion.

Treatment options are same as that for non HIV infected patients, however, there is more propensity of:

- Treatment failure
- Relapse
- Resistance to penicillin has been detected recently.

CSF examination is recommended if:

- There is eye involvement
- Treatment failure is suspected

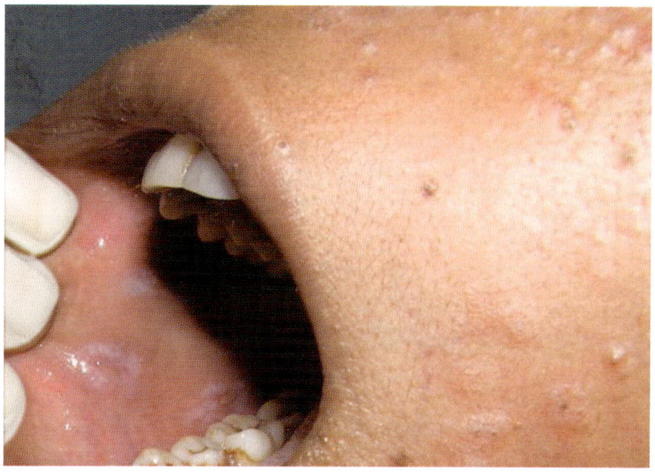

Fig. 4.38: Mucous patch in a patient with secondary syphilis

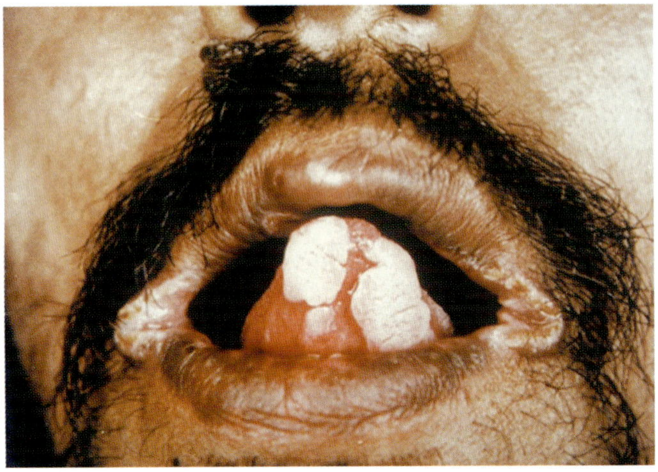

Fig. 4.39: Oral condyloma lata and split papules

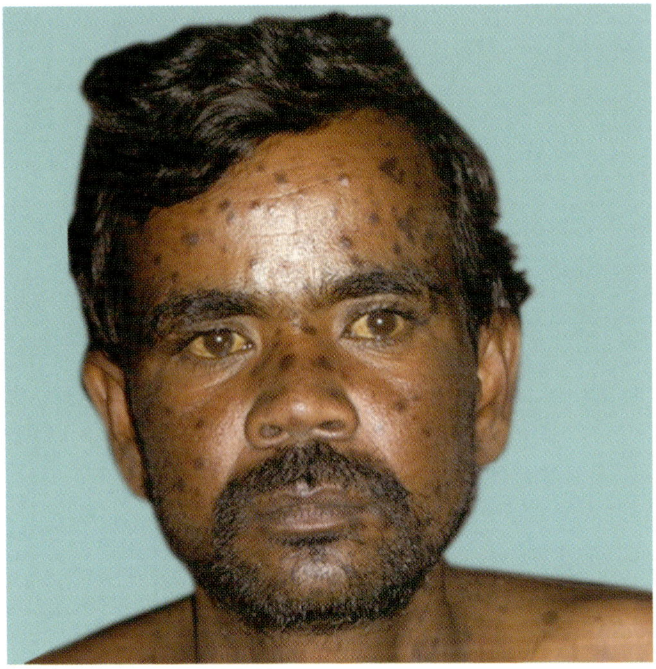

Fig. 4.40: Papulosquamous syphilides

- Relapse is seen
- Patient has been treated with any other regimen.

OTHER STIs

Various STIs, like cervicitis, vaginits, gonorrhea (Figs 4.44 and 4.45), urethritis, PID, etc. which are seen in our daily

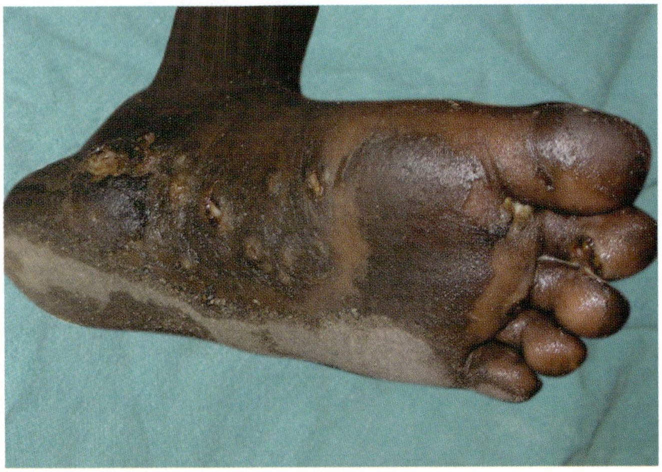

Fig. 4.41: Lues maligna in the same patient

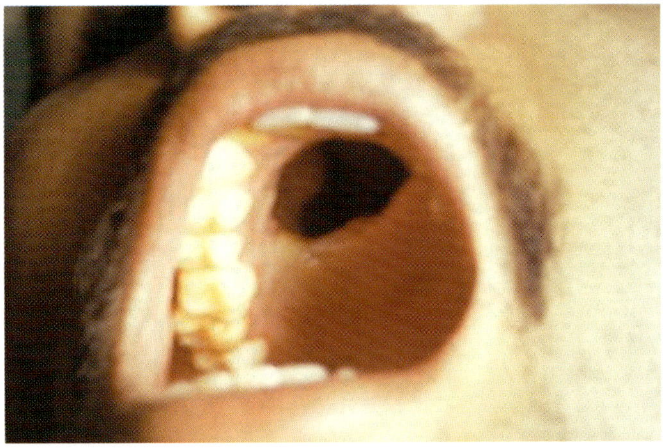

Fig. 4.42: Palatal perforation—tertiary syphilis

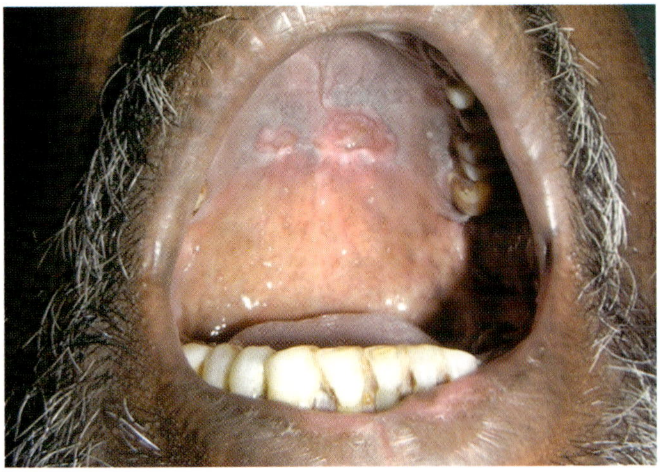

Fig. 4.43: Follow-up of a patient with gummata of tertiary syphilis; picture showing healing lesion after giving crystalline penicillin

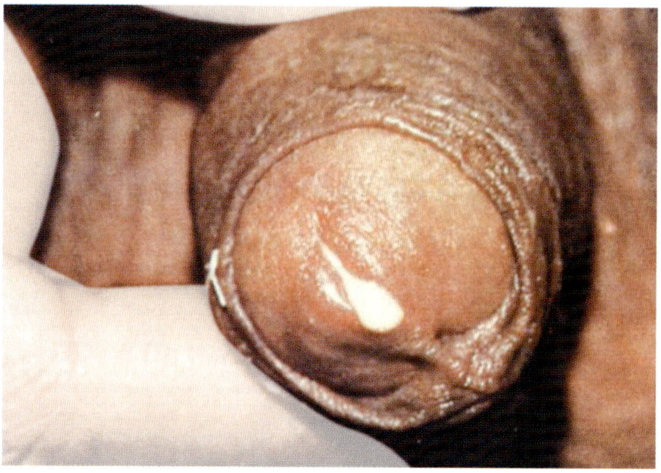

Fig. 4.44: Typical purulent discharge per urethra-gonorrhea

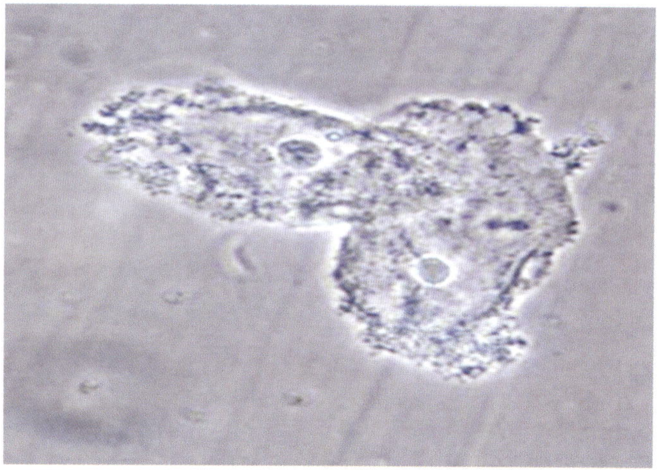

Fig. 4.46: Photograph showing clue cells—a simple OPD based diagnostic test for bacterial vaginosis (*Source* : CDC PHIL)

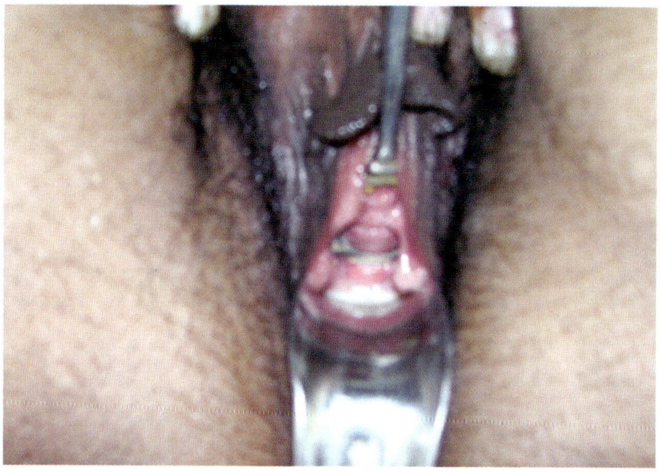

Fig. 4.45: Cervical discharge in a seroreactive female patient. Gram's stain showed presence of gram negative diplococci

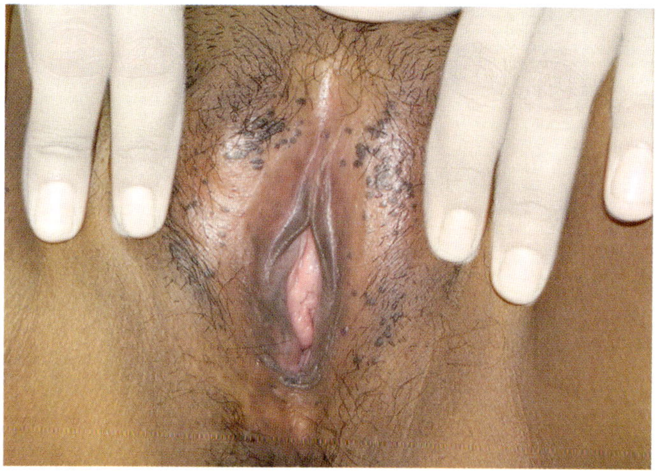

Fig. 4.47: Bowenoid papulosis in a female patient

practice have also been with the concurrent infection of HIV. There is not much difference observed in the presentation and management of the same, however an HIV transmission is seen with trichomoniasis and bacterial vaginosis (Fig. 4.46). STIs presenting as discharge like vaginits, cervicitis, urethritis, gonorrhea, NGU are equally implicated as a major risk factor for its who can acquire and transmit HIV.

5 NonInfectious Dermatosis in HIV/AIDS

A number of inflammatory noninfectious dermatoses have been found in HIV-infected patients. Only a few of these are related to presence of HIV. While in the other conditions, the exact mechanism and relationship to HIV is not known.

Most of these conditions vary in severity with the CD4 count (Figs 5.1 and 5.2).

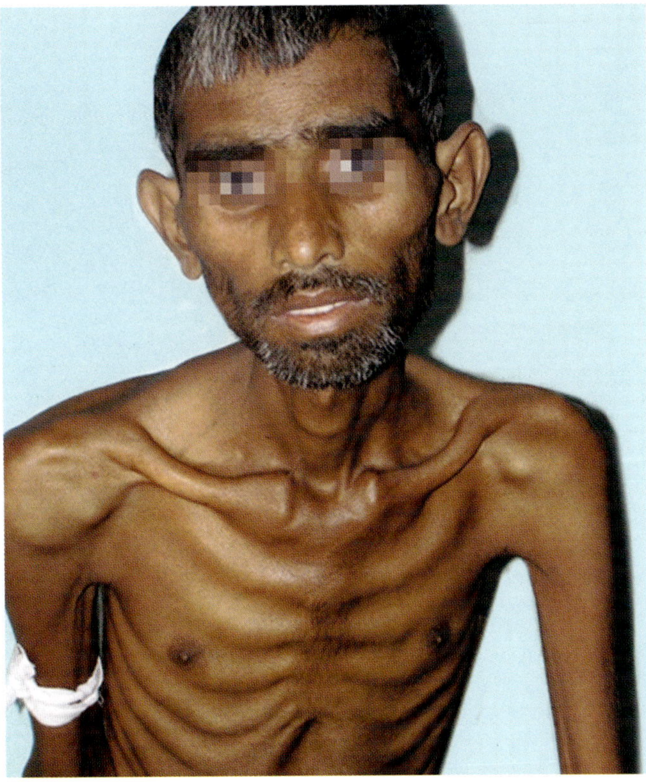

Fig. 5.1 Slim's disease

COMMON NONINFECTIOUS DERMATOSES IN HIV

- Pruritis
- Xerosis and icthyosis
- Seborrheic dermatitis
- Eosinophilic folliculitis
- Pruritic papular eruptions
- Drug eruptions
- Atopic dermatitis
- Psoriasis
- Reiters disease.

UNCOMMON DERMATOSES

- Photosensitivity
- Erythroderma

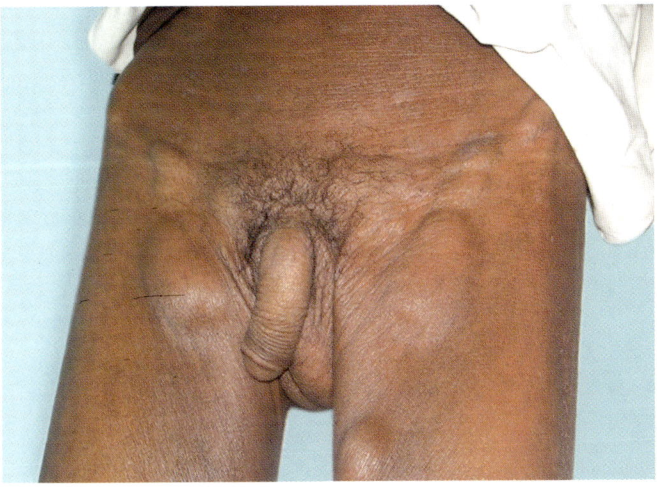

Fig. 5.2: Remarkable lymphadenopathy

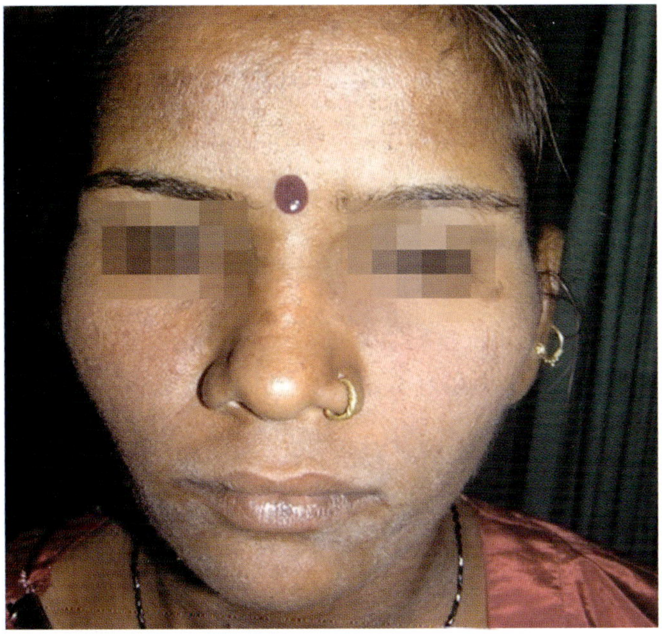

Fig. 5.3: A female patient with mild seborrheic dermatitis

- Allergic contact dermatitis
- Papuloerythroderma
- Persistent insect bite reaction
- Prurigo nodularis
- Pityriasis rubra pilaris
- Perforating folliculitis
- Urticaria
- Erythema nodosum
- Hidradenitis suppuritiva
- Deficiency dermatitis
- Cutaneous malignancies.

SEBORRHEIC DERMATITIS

As many as 85% of HIV-infected patients may have seborrheic dermatitis. It may be an indicator of seroconversion. Typically yellowish white greasy scales are present on an erythematous base. Most common sites include the scalp, face (Figs 5.3 and 5.4) especially the nasolabial folds, retroauricular ares, upper back,

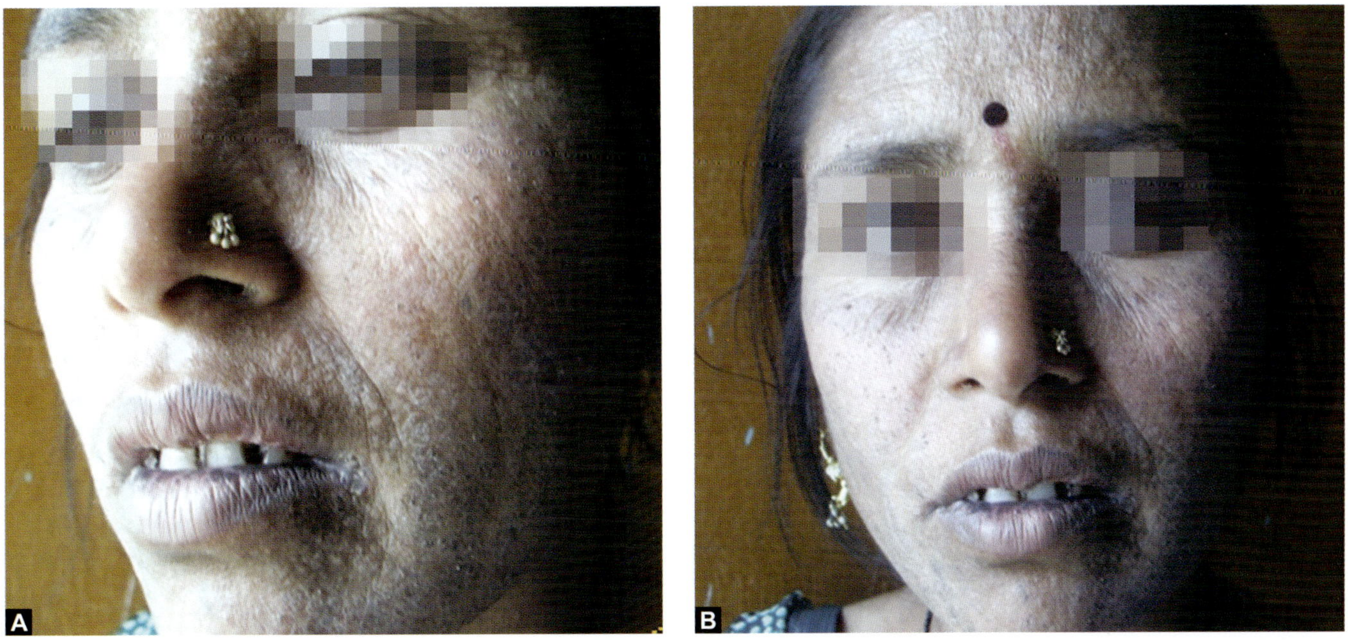

Figs 5.4A and B: Female patients with severe seborrheic dermatitis

chest and intertrigenous areas. Occasional patients present with erythroderma (Fig. 5.5).

It is resistant to most treatment. Mild cases may be managed with ketoconazole. For severe cases, topical steroids, ketoconazole shampoos, coal tar, salicylic acid and UVB may be tried. Refractory cases respond to highly active antiretroviral therapy (HAART) at times.

EOSINOPHILIC FOLLICULITIS

It is a common chronic pruritic condition occurring in HIV-infected people. There is a centripetal eruption of pruritic, erythematous perifollicular papules and rarely pustules over face and trunk . There may be secondary excoriation, pigmenten prurigo like changes (Figs 5.8 and 5.9).

Histology is characteristic with folliculocentric eosinophilic and lymphocytic infiltrate. Flame figures and eosinophilic abscesses may be seen. Treatment options include topical steroids, oral isotretinoin, oral itraconazole, anti-histamines, oral metronidazole and topical permethrin (5%). Phototherapy (UVA and UVB) is one of the most successful treatment option.

Diagnosis of this condition should be made after the other causes of papular pruritic eruption have been excluded.

PRURITIC PAPULAR ERUPTIONS

It is a common dermatoses affecting 15–45% of HIV infected patients. Etiology is not known. Multiple skin colored papules are seen symmetrically on the extremities, trunk and face (Figs 5.6 and 5.7). It is a diagnosis of exclusion.

Differential diagnosis includes demodex folliculitis, eosinophilic folliculitis, scabies, staphylococcal folliculitis, papular urticaria and pityrosporum folliculitis. Treatment includes topical steroids, oral antibiotics, emollients, anti-histamines, oral and topical permethrin (5%). Pentoxiphylline and thalidomide have been effective in few cases.

PSORIASIS

The incidence of psoriasis in HIV-infected patients does not seem to be increased or only marginally increased but HIV appears to alters the course of disease (Figs 5.10 to 5.12 and 5.14 to 5.16).

More than one type of morphological variants may occur in the same patient. Incidence of psoriatic arthritis is higher (Figs 5.13, 5.18 and 5.19). Treatment remains the same as in immunocompetent patients. Methotrexate and ciclosporin should be avoided due to risk of immunosuppression.

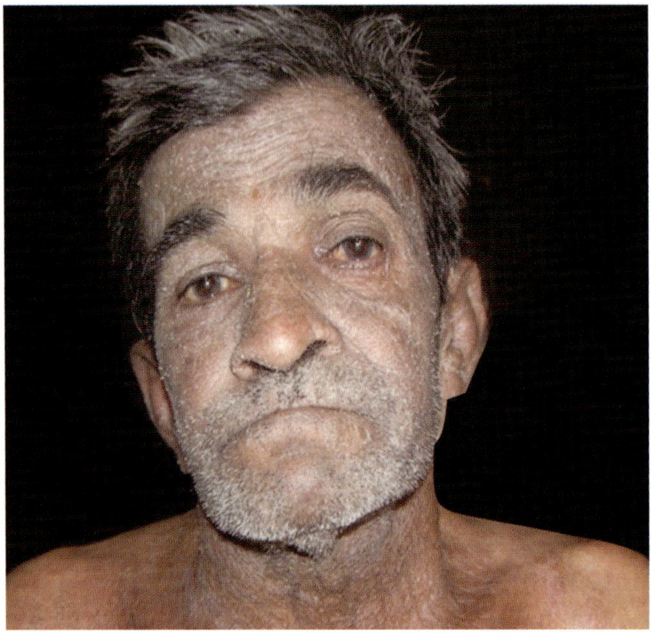

Fig 5.5: Severe seborrheic dermatitis. Patient later developed erythroderma

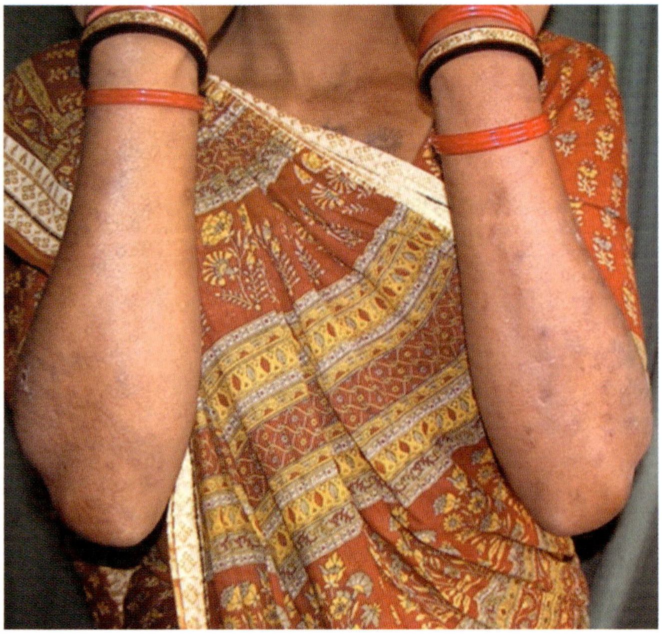

Fig. 5.6: Pruritic papular of HIV over forearm

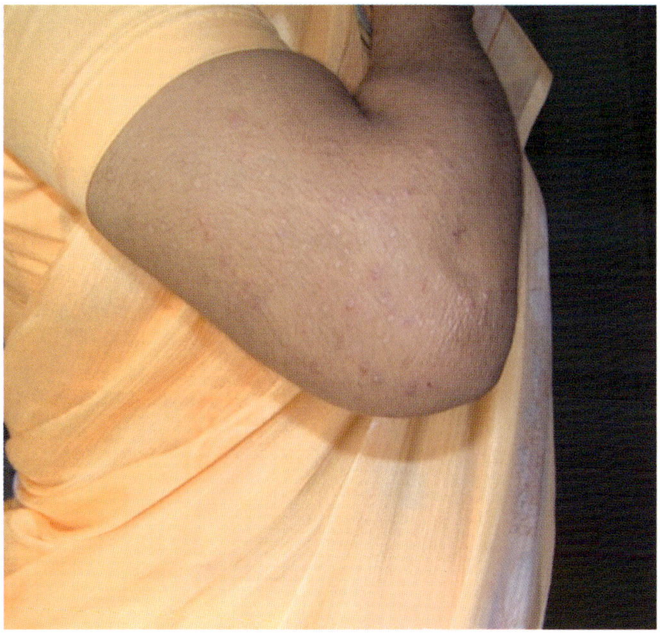

Fig. 5.7: Pruritic papular eruptions

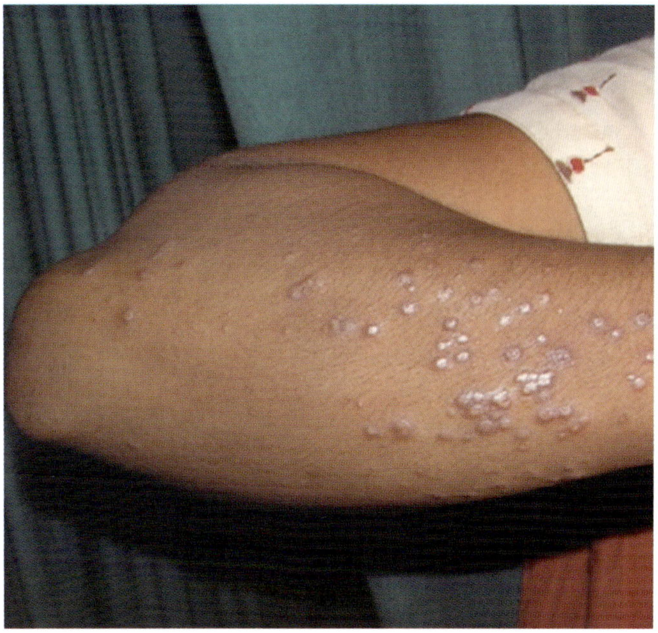

Fig. 5.9: Papular eruptions of eosinophilic folliculities

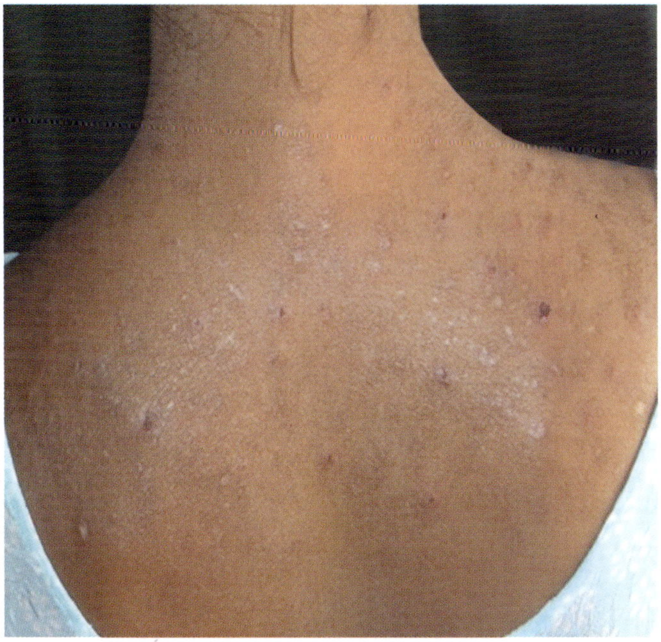

Fig. 5.8: Follicular papules over back of a female with eosinophilic folliculitis

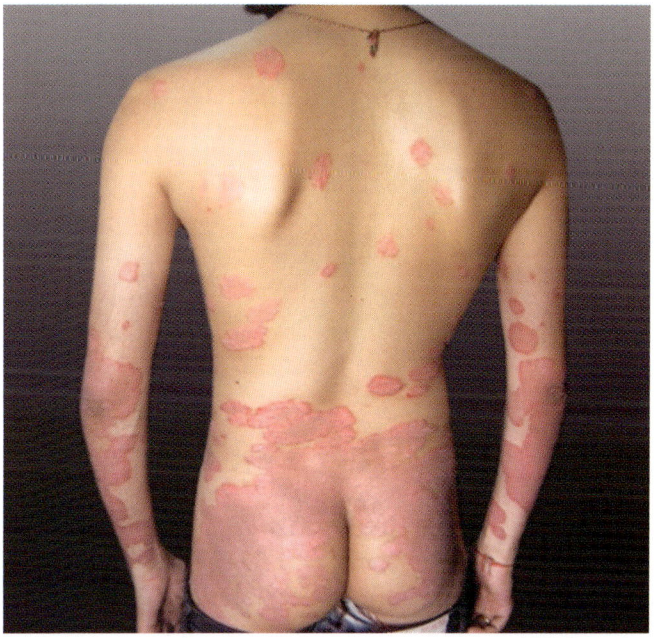

Fig. 5.10: Chronic plaque psoriasis

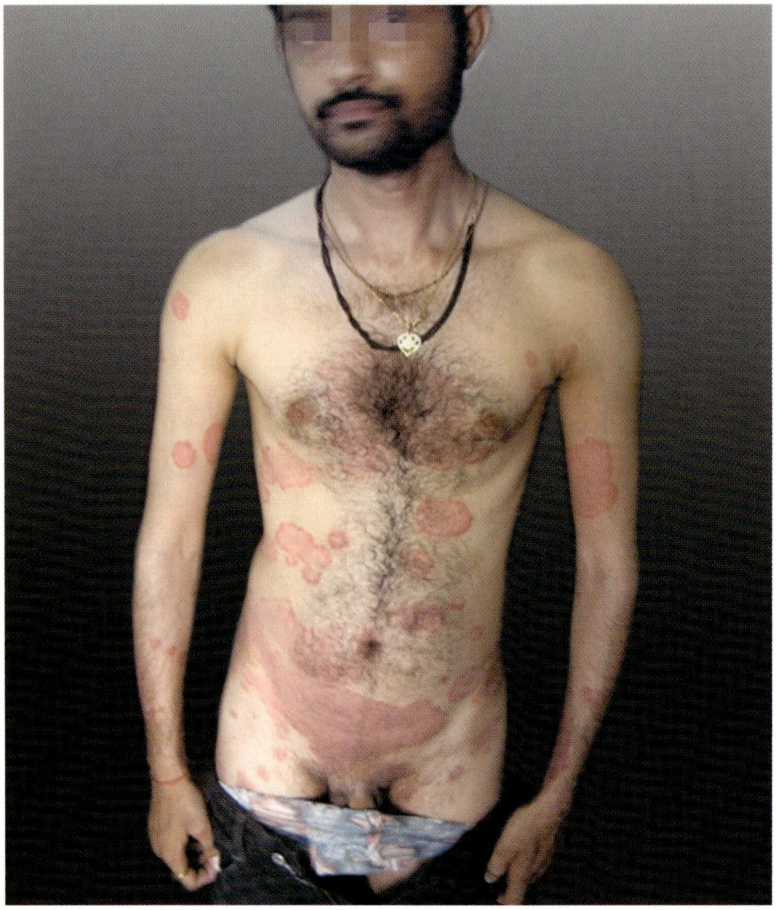

Fig. 5.11: Erythrodermic psoriasis

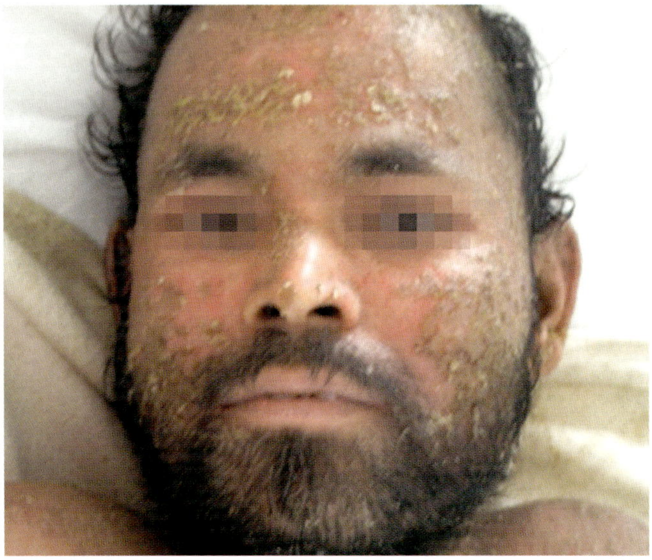

Fig. 5.12: Facial and enytheme scaling in a case of psoriasis erythroderma

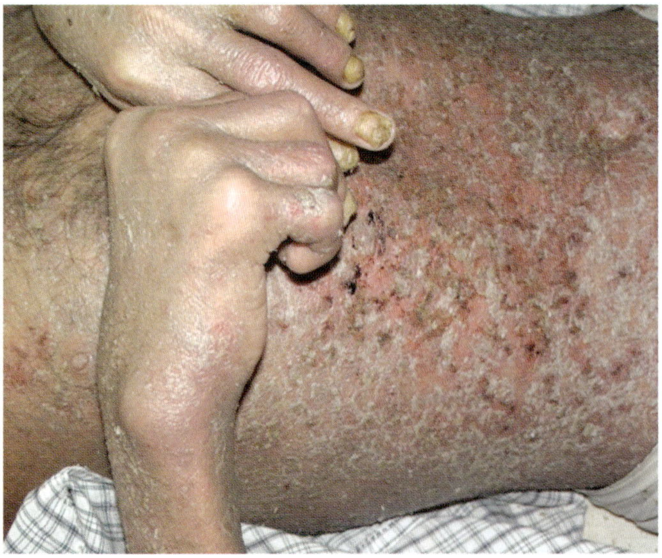

Fig. 5.13: Psoriatic arthropathy in the same patient along with involvement trunk

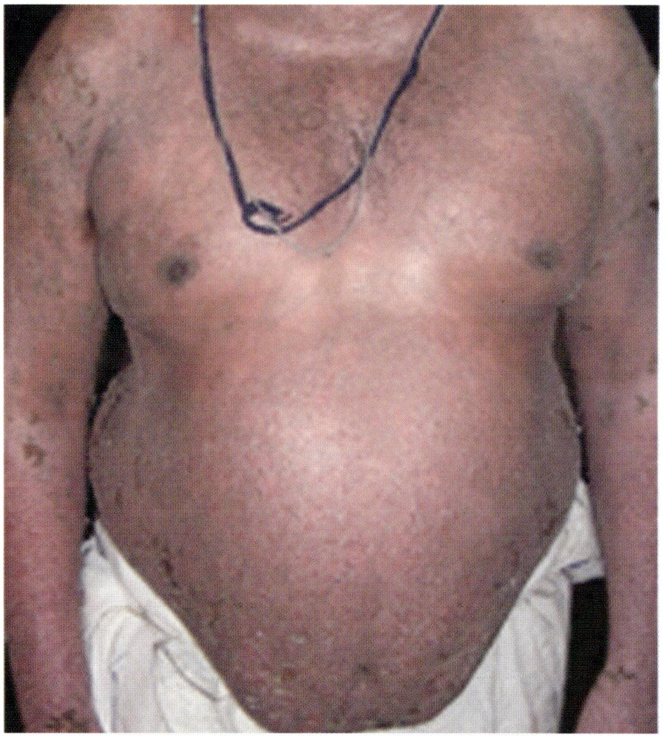

Fig. 5.14: Psoriatic erythroderma

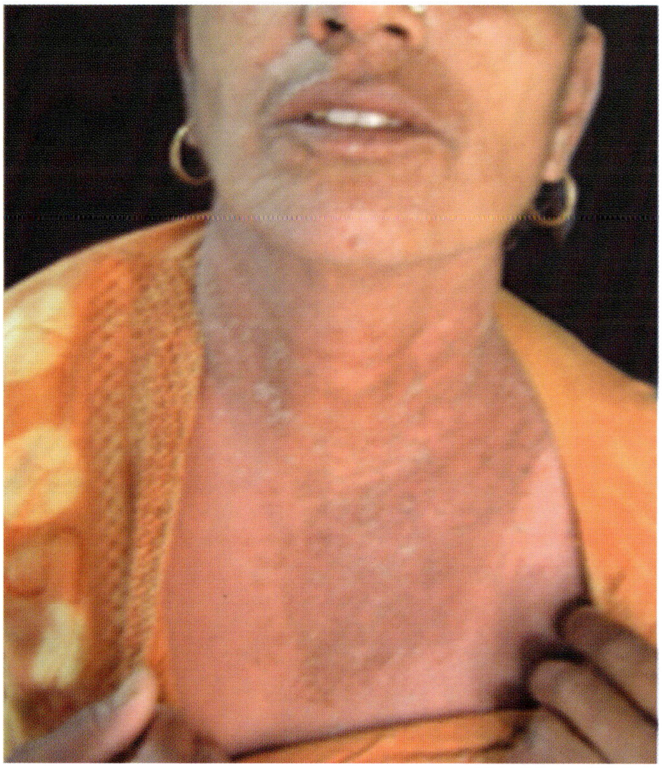

Fig. 5.15: Pustular psoriasis in a female patient

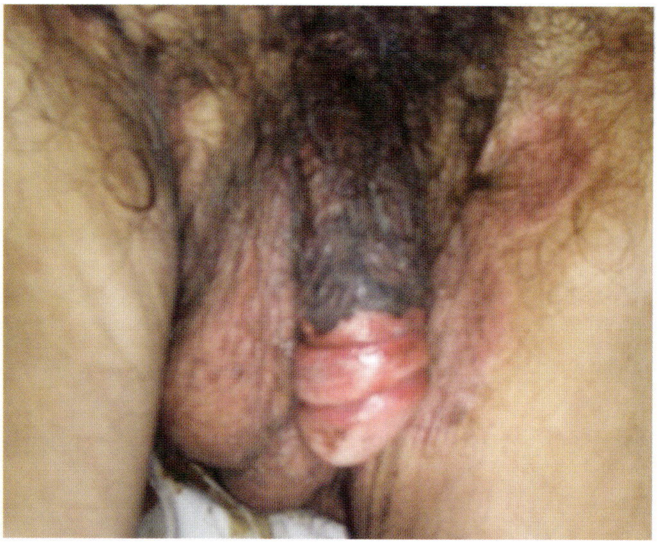

Fig. 5.16: Circinate balanitis in the same patient as in Fig. 5.19

REITER'S DISEASE

It is characterized by a triad of conjunctivitis, urethritis and arthritis of more than one month duration. The arthritis is more frequent and incapaciating in these patients (Figs 5.17A and B):

Subacute Cutaneous Lupus Erythematosus (SCLE) (Refer Figures 5.20A and B)

PHOTOSENSITIVITY

An increased incidence of photosensitivity is found with HIV,the etiology of which is poorly understood. Use of phototoxic drugs may be responsible (Figs 5.20 to 5.22 and 5.29 to 5.31).

OTHER RARE ASSOCIATIONS WITH HIV

Hidradenitis Suppuritiva

It is a chronic, recurrent disease affecting the apocrine gland bearing areas (axilla, groin) (Figs 5.23 to 5.25) due to occlusion of these glands. Clinically it is characterized by abscesses and sinus formation in these areas.

Granuloma Annulare

This is characterized by papular or annular, generalized skin lesion (Fig. 5.32).

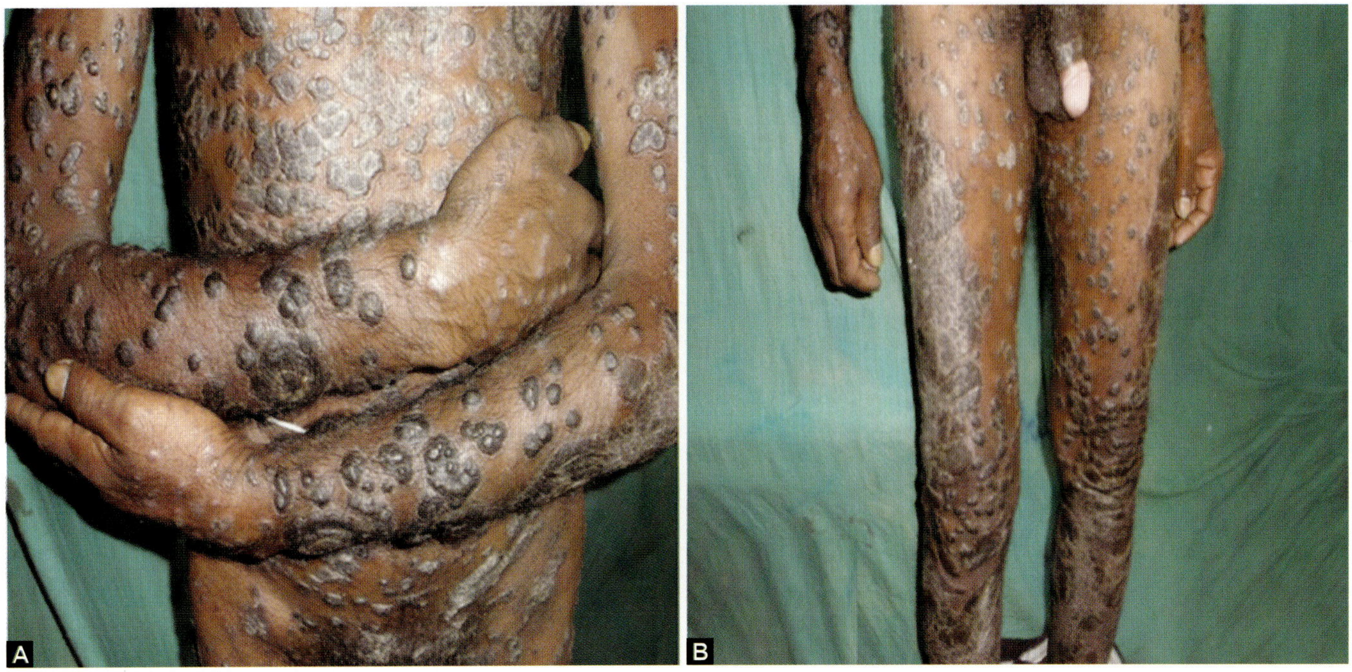

Figs 5.17A and B: Reiter's disease-lesions over Body

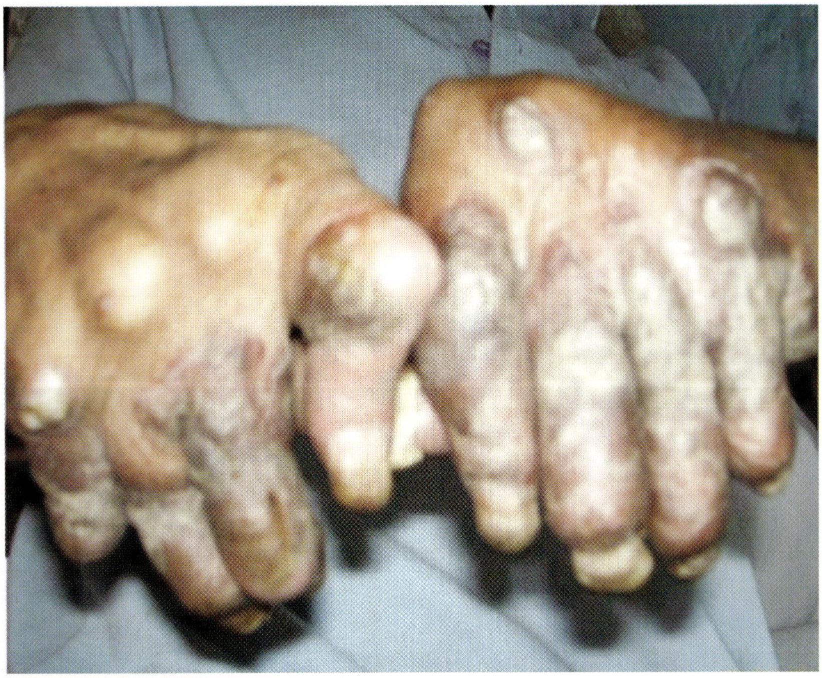

Fig. 5.18: Psoriatic arthropathy involving hand joints

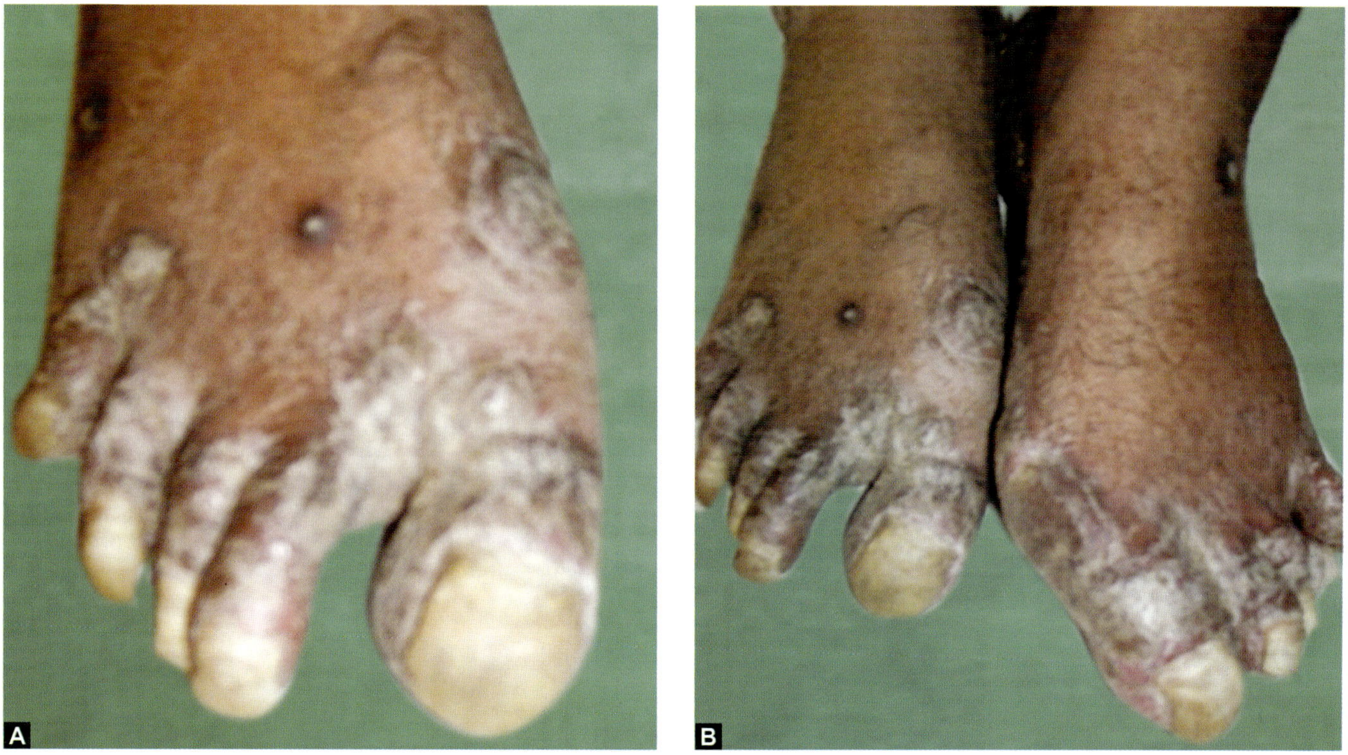

Figs 5.19A and B: Severe arthropathy

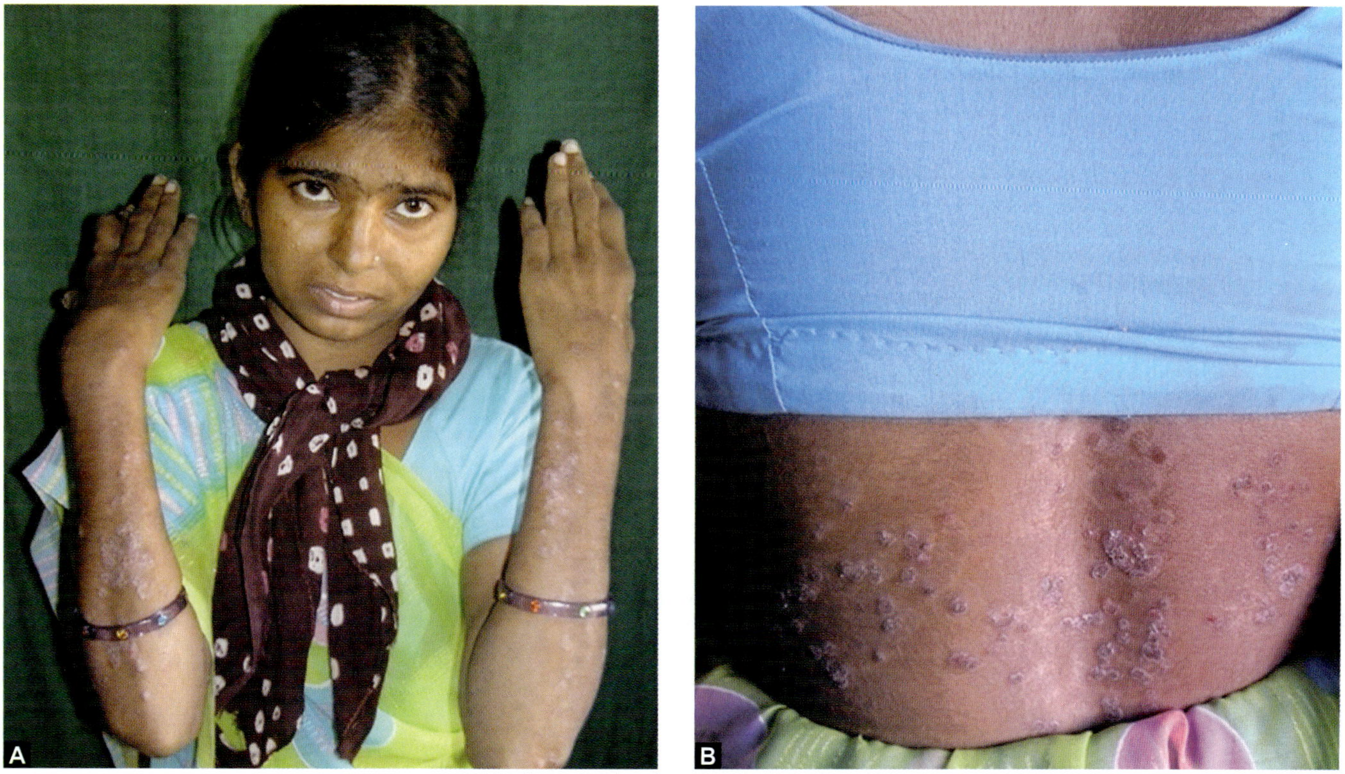

Figs 5.20A and B: Typical papulosquamous lesions seen in female with SCLE

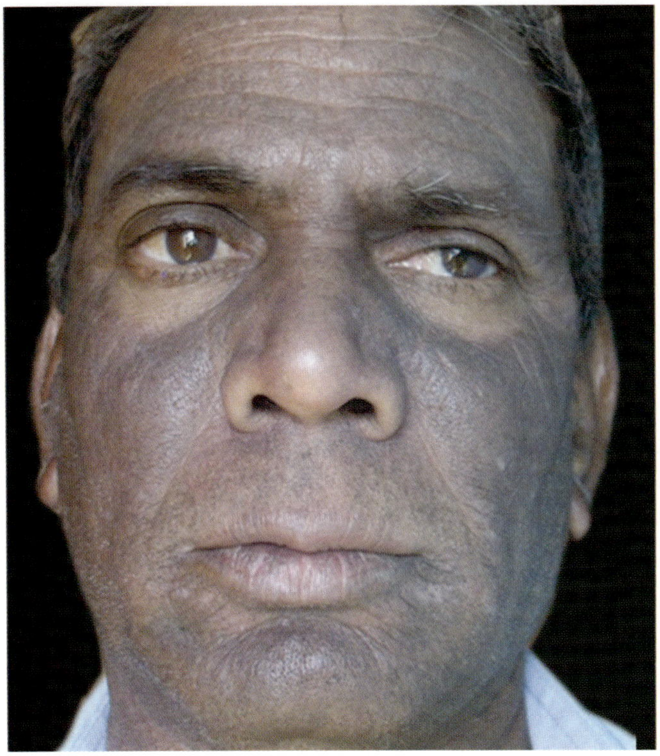

Fig. 5.21: Photosensitivity in patient who was on TMP-SMZ prophylaxis

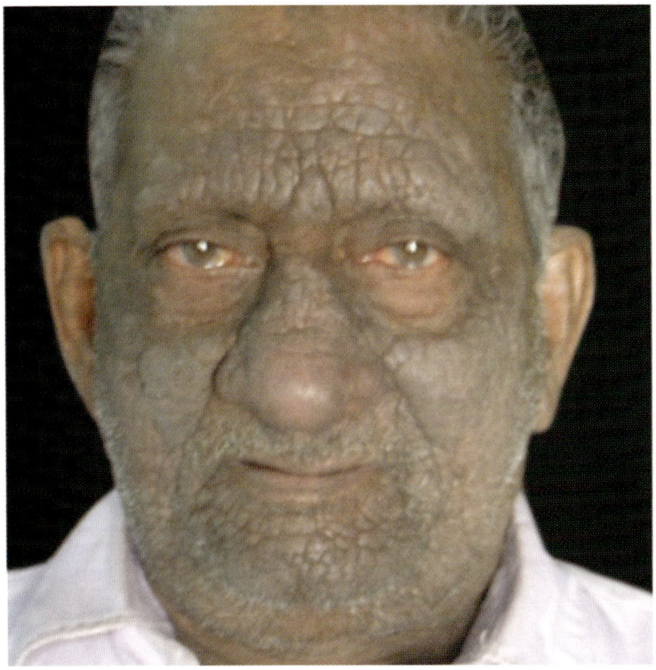

Fig. 5.22: Chronic actinic dermatitis with hyperpigmentation, scaling and lichenification of exposed areas

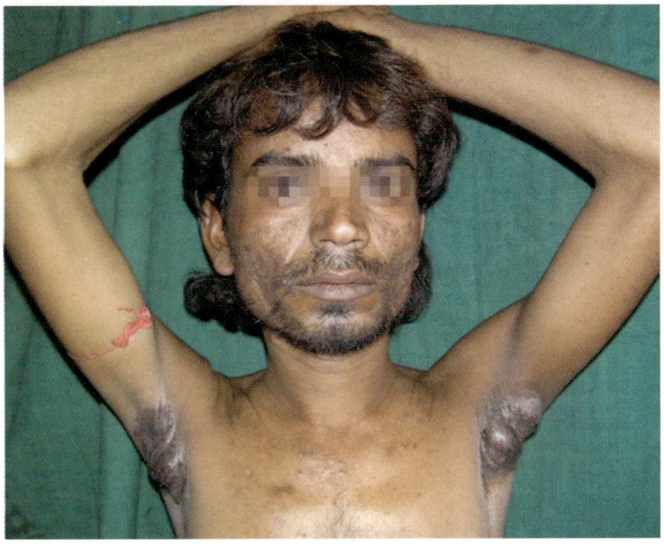

Fig. 5.23: Multiple abscesses in axilla-a case of hidradenitis suppurativa

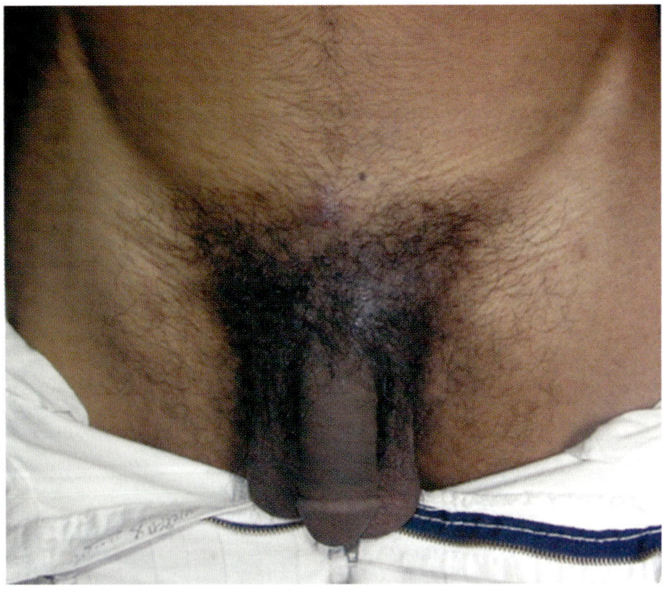

Fig. 5.24: Hidradenitis suppurativa involving groins

Trichomegaly

Trichomegaly appears to be particularly common, especially in pediatric patients. What causes trichomegaly still remains unknown (Fig. 5.26).

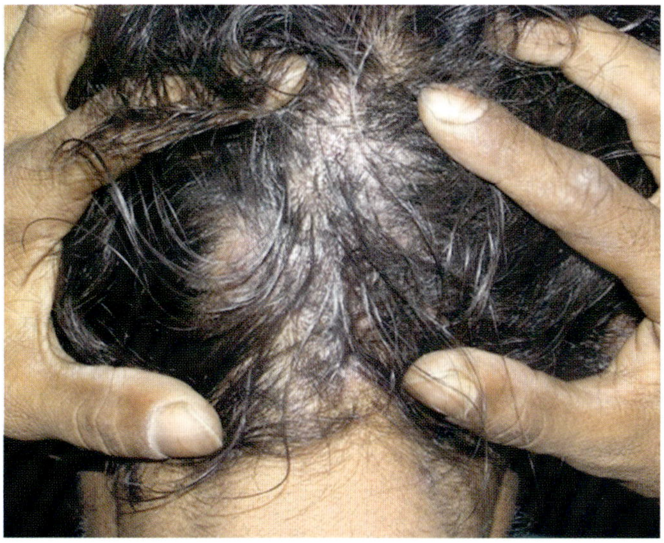

Fig. 5.25: Folliculitis of scalp in same patient in Figures 5.23 and 5.24

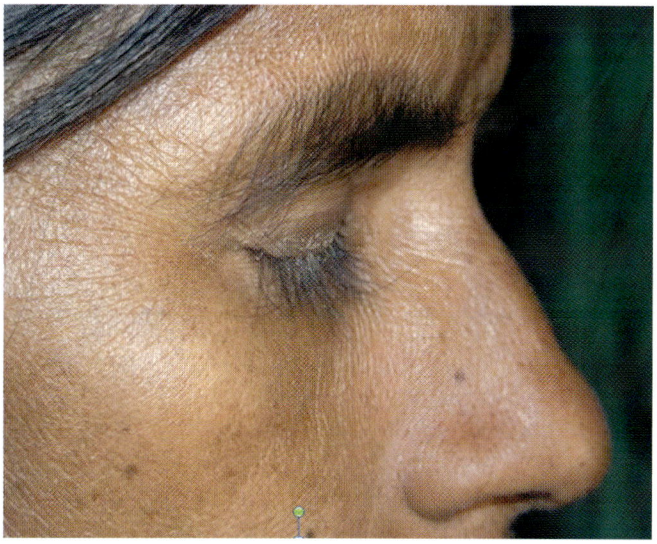

Fig. 5.26: Adult patient with trichomegaly

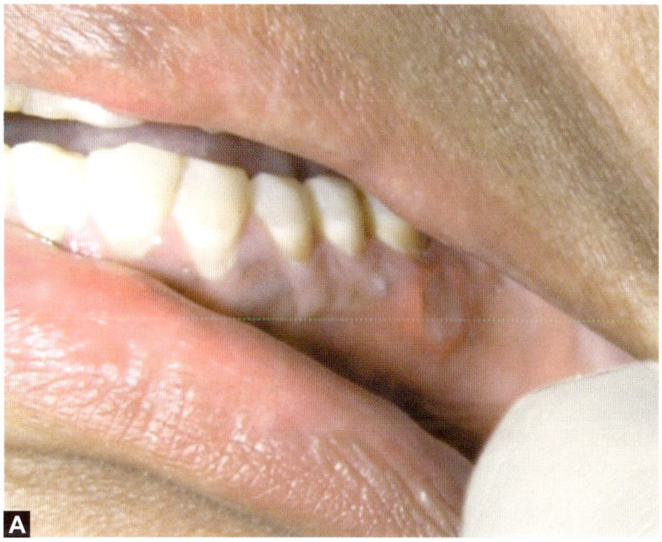

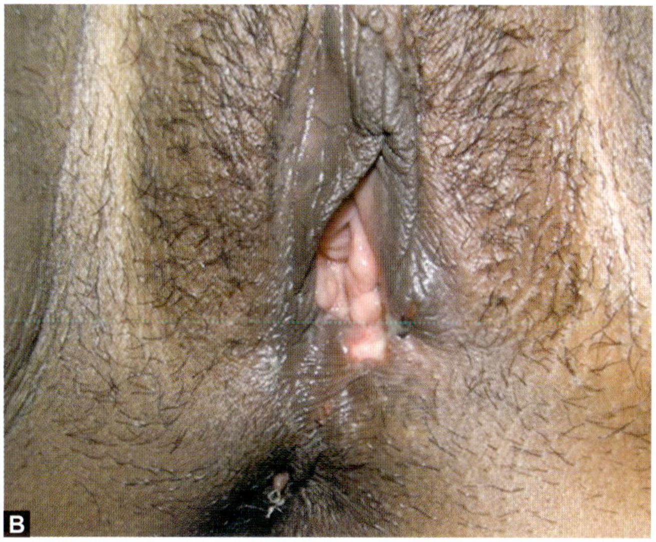

Figs 5.27A and B: Oral and genital aphthae in a patient with Behçet's disease

BEHÇET'S SYNDROME

HIV-infected patients are (Figs 5.27A and B) patients generally presents with recurrent oral and genital ulceration.

NEOPLASMS

Incidence of certain malignancies appears to be increased in HIV-infected patients (Fig. 5.28). These include Kaposi's sarcoma (Fig. 5.33), lymphoma and squamous cell carcinoma.

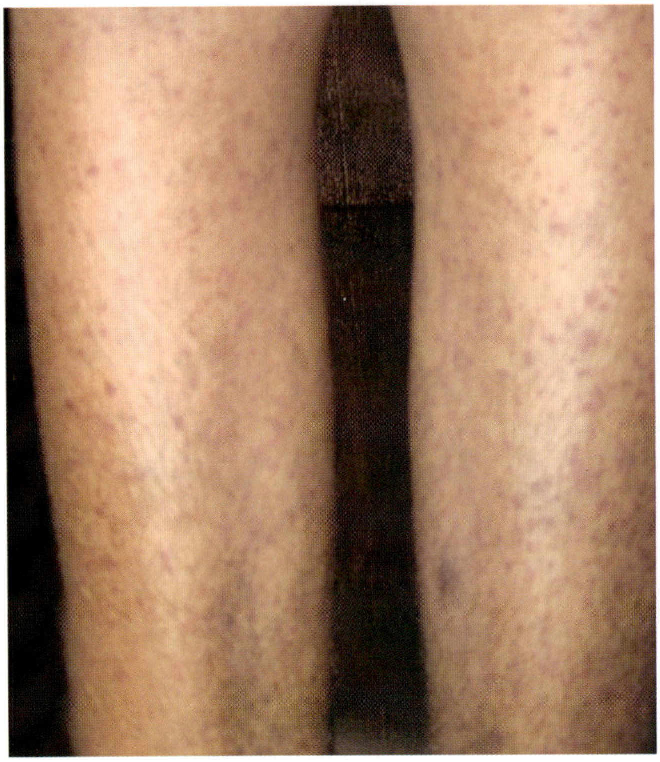

Fig. 5.28: Henoch Schonlein purpura

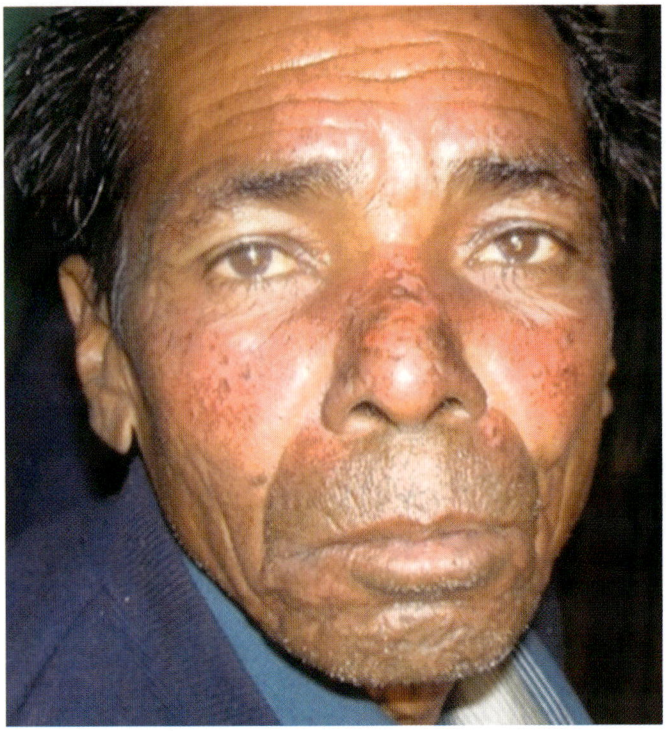

Fig 5.30: Dermatitis affecting photoexposed areas in this patient with Pellagra

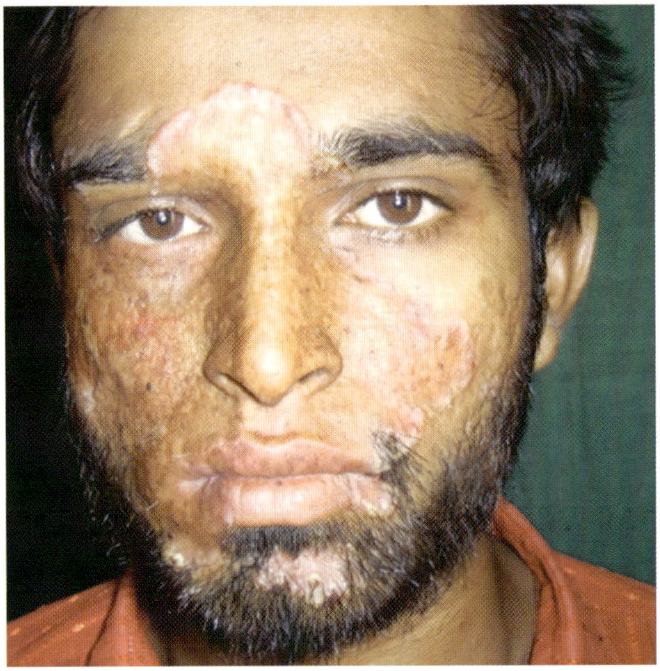

Fig 5.29: Porokeratosis of Mibelli-a rare association

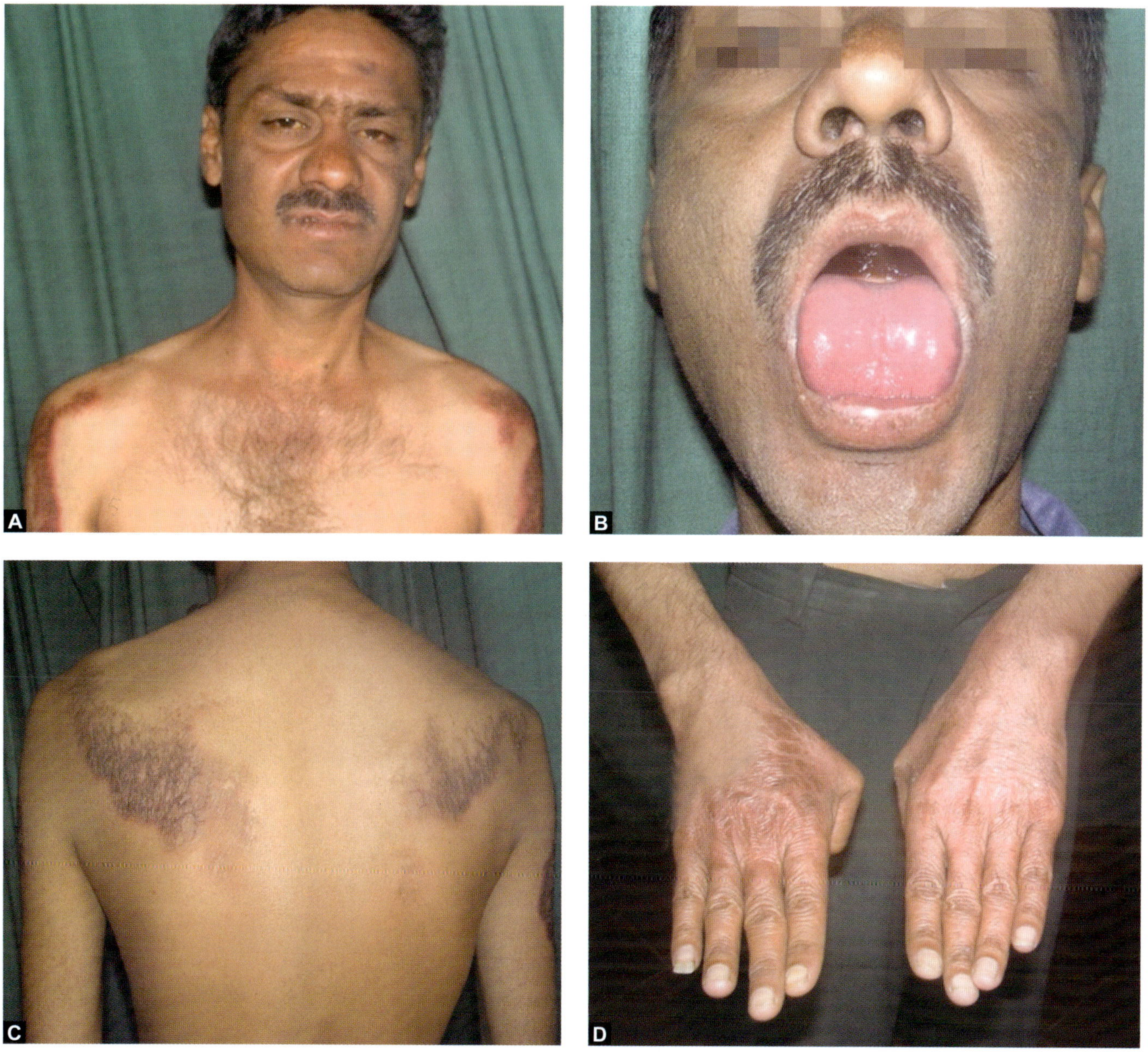

Figs 5.31A to D: Pellagra dermatitis with glossitis

Kaposi's Sarcoma

It is caused by HHV-8. It is rare in India. Lesions appear as erythematous macules or papules and later increase in size to form violaceous nodules and plaques (Fig. 5.33). Most common sites involved are the trunk, legs, face and oral cavity.

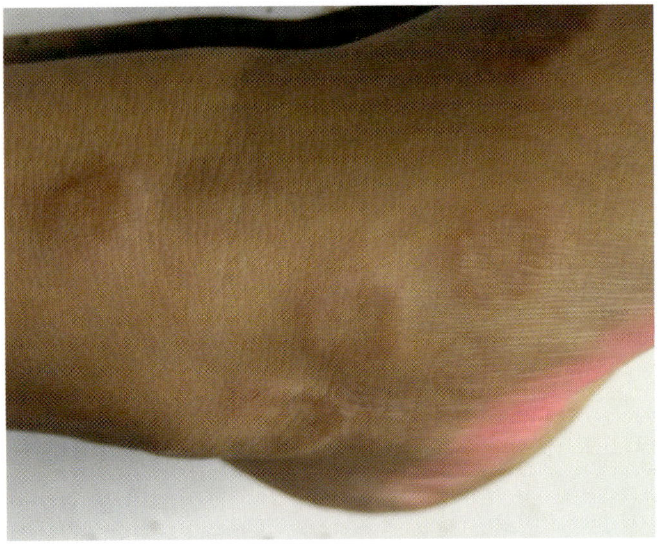

Fig 5.32: Granuloma annulare

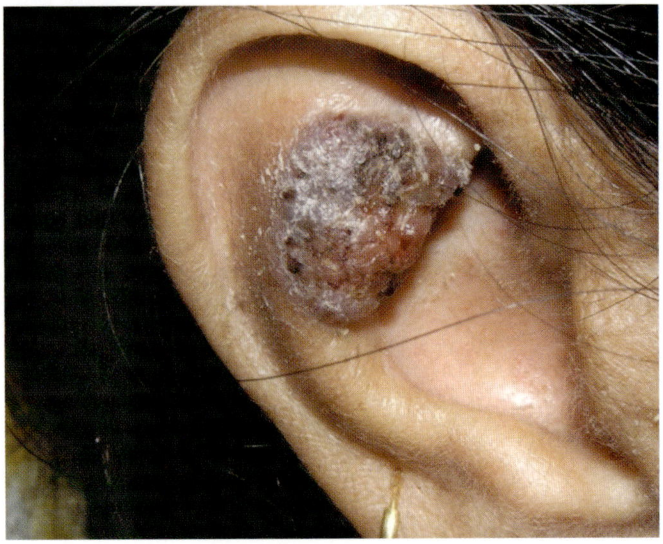

Fig. 5.34: Squamous cell carcinoma

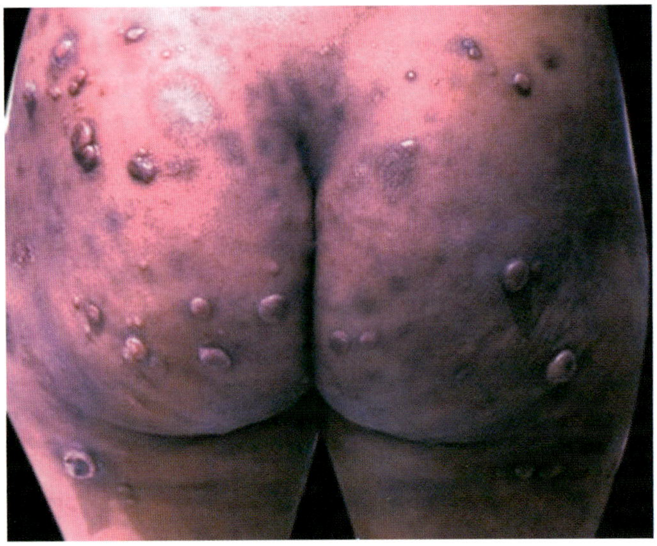

Fig. 5.33: Kaposi sarcoma

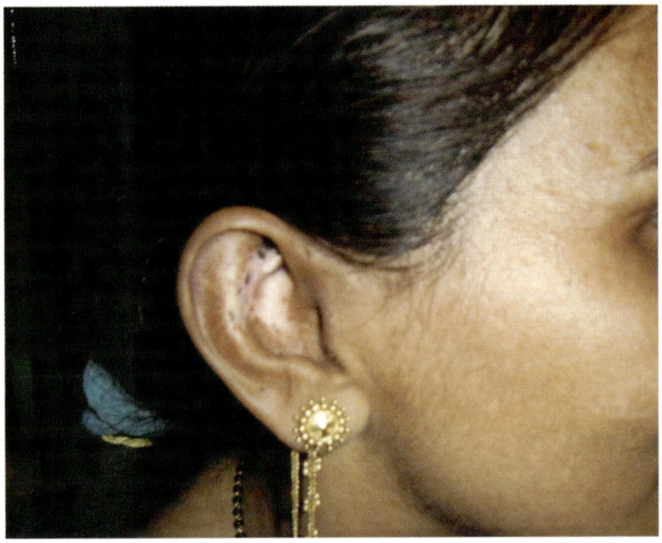

Fig. 5.35: SCC—postexcision and radiotherapy

Squamous Cell Carcinoma (Figs 5.34 to 5.37)

It presents as verrucous growth or asymptomatic ulcer with rolled out edges. Treatment consists of surgical excision or radiation therapy.

B-cell Lymphoma

Primary cutaneous lymphomas are rare diseases counting for less than 24% of all cutaneous lymphoma (Fig. 5.38).

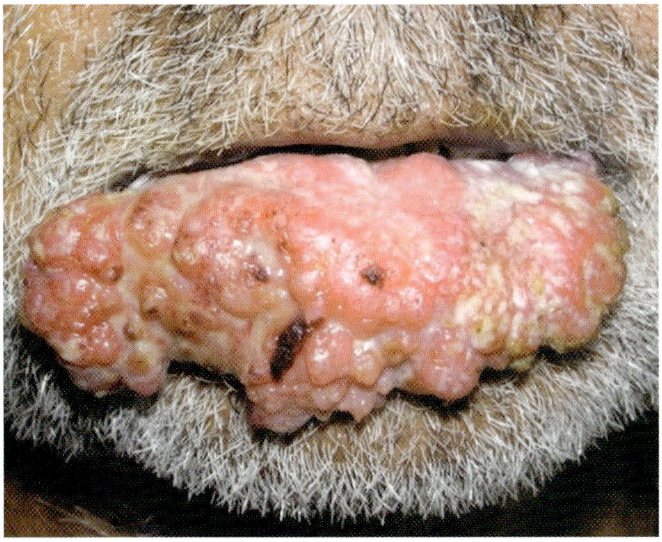

Fig. 5.36: Squamous cell carcinoma of lip

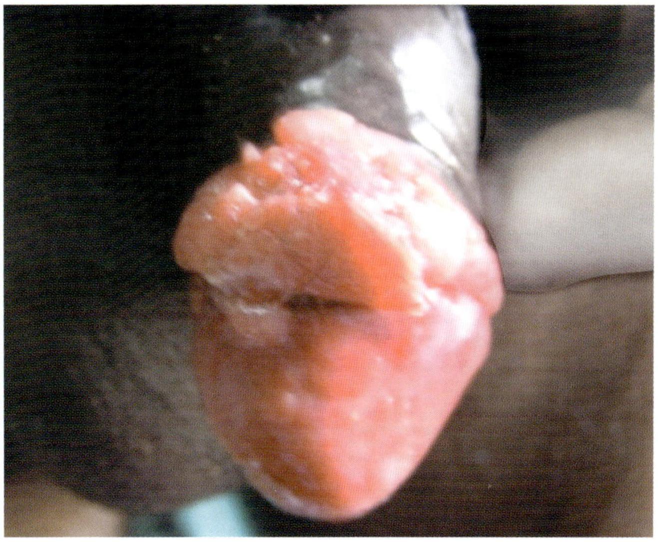

Fig. 5.37: Squamous cell carcinoma—penis

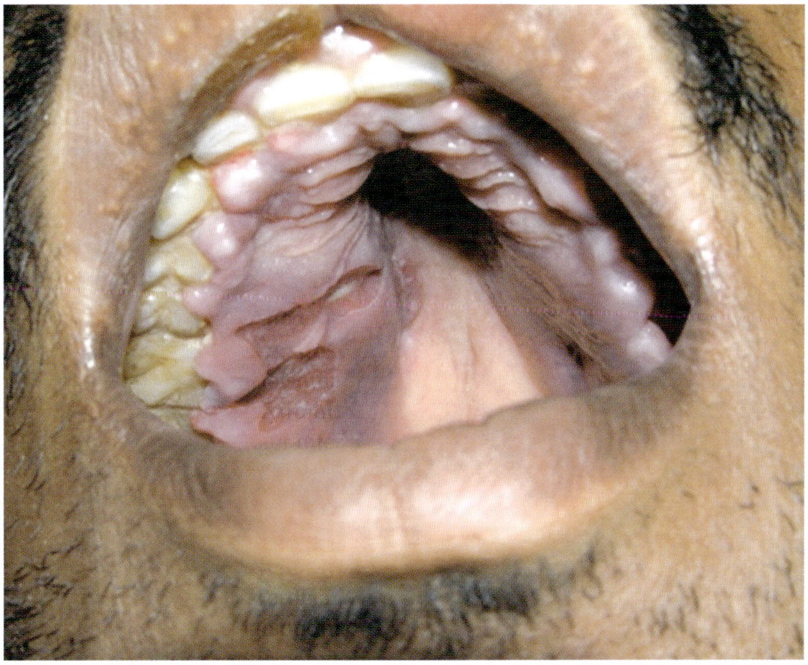

Fig. 5.38: Oral lesion in B-cell lymphoma

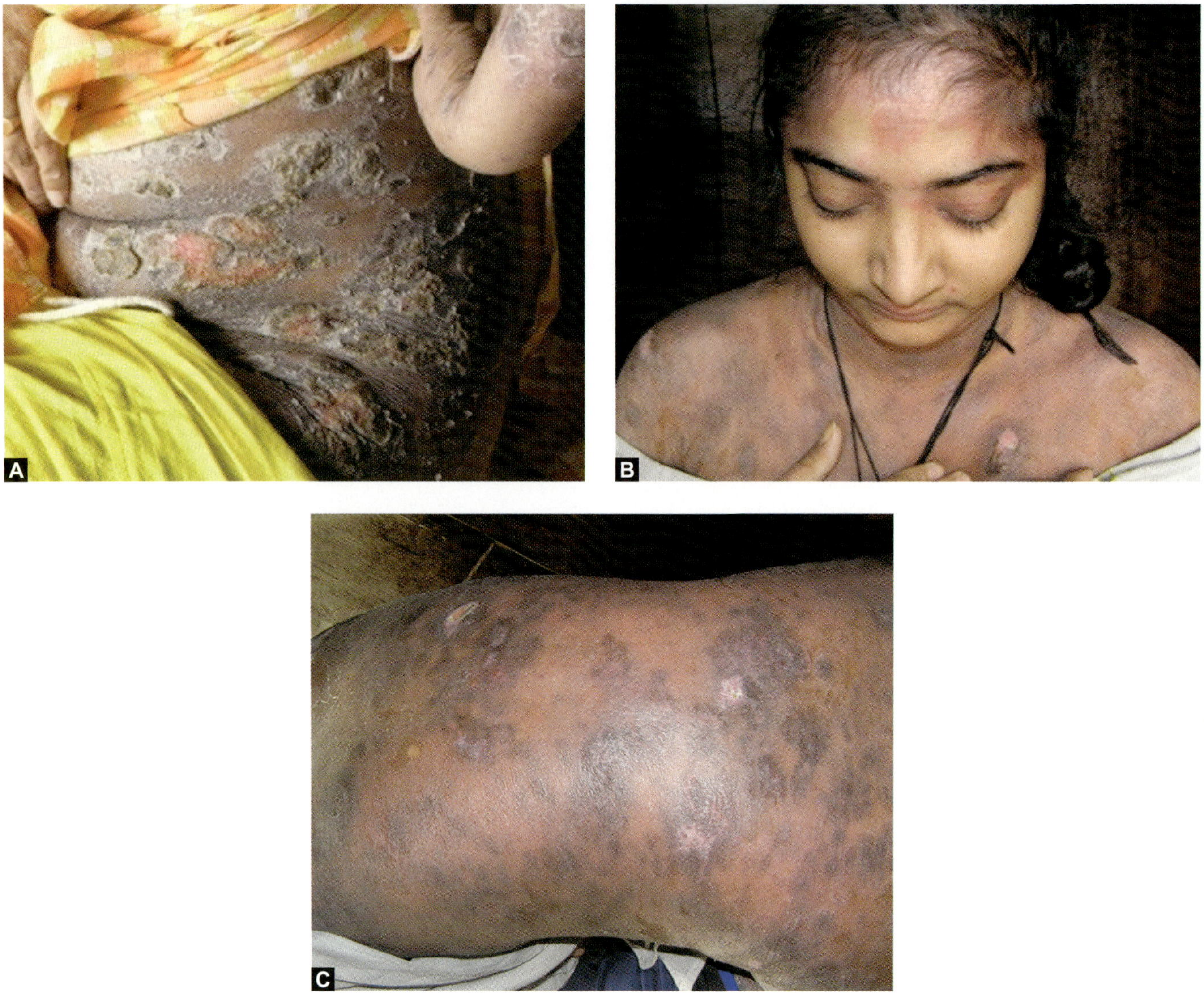

Figs 5.39A to C: T-cell lymphoma

T- Cell Lymphoma

The skin is infiltrated with T lymphocytes, usually a disease seen in middle aged or elderly people. Various morphological forms are seen. Lymphnodes, bone marrow evaluation will help to stage the disease (Figs 5.39A to C).

6 Oral Cavity

One finger in the mouth and one finger in the rectum makes a good clinician.

—Sir William Osler

- In respect to the development, structure, microbiology, function and diseases, the oral cavity has its own position in human body
- The mucosa of oral cavity is of much importance for dermatologist's point of view as it is developed from ectoderm
- Diseases in oral cavity can be classified as :
  1. Infectious diseases
  2. Non infectious diseases
  3. Drug induced reactions
  4. Malignant conditions
- Structures, which can be involved in disease process include peridontium, gingiva, oral mucosa, hard palate, soft palate, tonsils, lips, etc.

INFECTIOUS DISEASES

A. *Acute necrotizing (ulcerating) gingivitis*
   Synonyms: Vincent's infection
   - It is a rapidly progressive ulceration caused by normal commensals of the oral cavity it becomes pathogenic when local resistance is reduced, typically starting at the tip of interdental papilla, spreading along with gingival margins and going on to cause acute destruction of the periodontal tissue high has been seen in incidence HIV patients
   - Anaerobic fusiform bacteria and spirochetes are implicated
   - Acute onset of gingival soreness and bleeding along with halitosis is characteristic feature in children between the ages of 3 years and 10 years.

B. *Gingival ulcers*: They can occur in HIV patient.

C. *Tuberculosis*: Mycobacterial oral ulcers caused by mycobacterium avium intracellular having reported as a complication of AIDS.

D. Herpes simplex
   - HSV-1 causes primary herpetic stomatitis and recurrent herpes labialis (Fig. 6.1)
   - Oral infection with HSV-2 is frequently seen as orogenital sex practices are more frequent these days
   - Primary herpetic gingivostomatitis (Fig. 6.2) is the most common form of stomatitis in children, manifests with prodromal symptoms of high fever, headache and anterior cervical lymphadenopathy

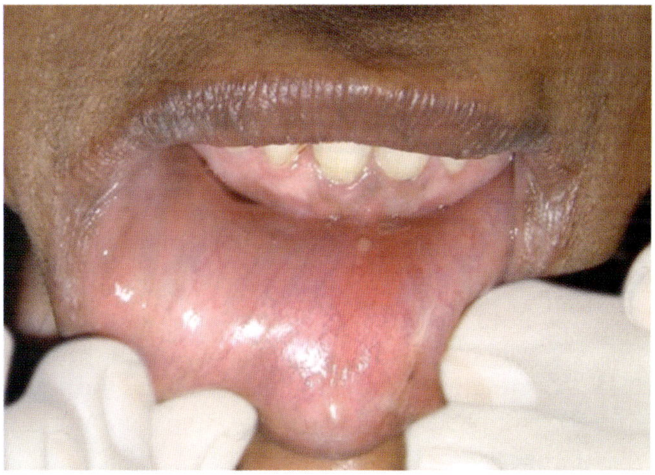

Fig. 6.1: Herpetic ulcer over lower lip mucosa with perilesional erythema

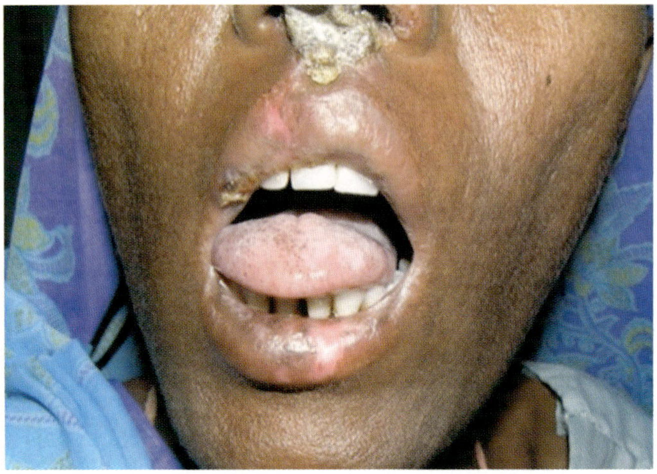

Fig. 6.2: Extensive herpes labialis

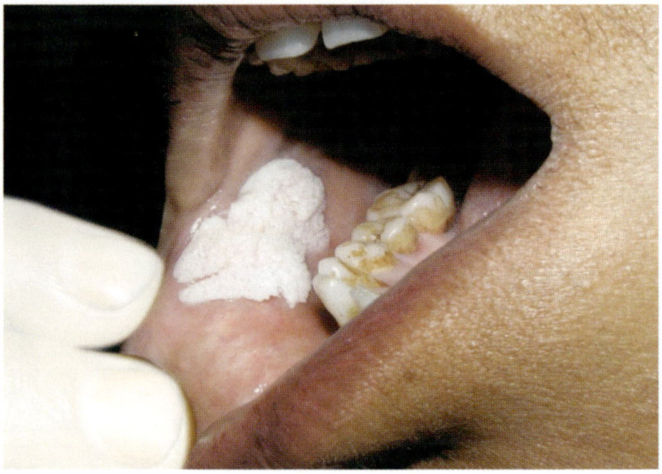

Fig. 6.4: Wart on buccal mucosa

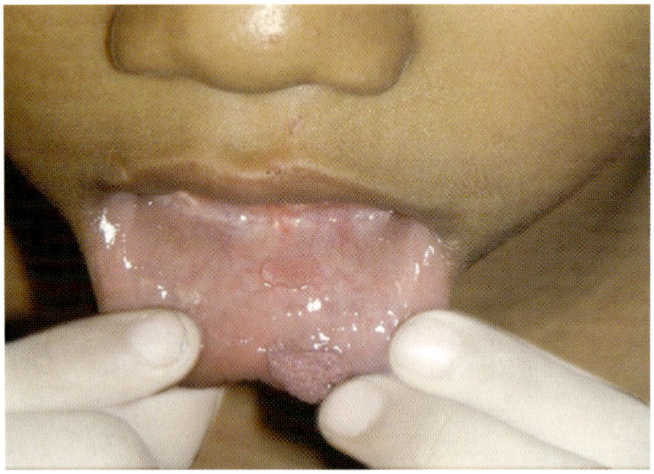

Fig. 6.3: Wart on lower lip of child

- Antiviral drugs can be used in severe stomatitis and in immunocompromised patients.

E. Herpes zoster
- Third most common cutaneous manifestation of HIV can also occur in oral cavity
- It appears as grouped vesicles on buccal mucosa, tongue, palate and gingiva unilaterally distributed along the area supplied by maxillary and mandibular division of trigeminal nerve
- If geniculate ganglion is involved Ramsay-Hunt syndrome occurs, which is characterized by unilateral facial plasy with vesicles in the ipsilateral ear and ulcers in ipsilateral soft palate.

F. *Warts* :They can be seen in oral cavity in HIV positive individual (Figs 6.3 and 6.4).

G. Molluscum contagiosum
- It is clinical sign of marked HIV progression and very low CD4 count
- Widespread infection on the face (Fig. 6.5) in form of giant molluscum is highly characteristic of late HIV disease
- Atypical molluscum contagiosum is also common in HIV patients often require biopsy for diagnosis.

H. Oral hairy leukoplakia
- This condition caused by Epstein Barr virus, manifests as a slightly raised white corrugated plaque on lateral aspect of tongue of HIV patients (Figs 6.6 and 6.7)
- It is highly suggestive of AIDS.

I. Kaposi's sarcoma
- It is an angioproliferative disorder caused by HHV-8
- Kaposi's sarcoma (KS) of the oral cavity is often associated with KS at other sites and sometimes, may be first manifestation of AIDS
- It has a marked predilection for homosexual or bisexual males

- Palate is the most common oral site for KS
- Early lesions appear as red or blue colored plaques (Fig. 6.8).

J. Candidiasis

- It is the most common opportunistic infection in patients with HIV as many as 90% with CD4 > 500
- Pathogenic species are candida albicans, candida dubiliniensis
- It manifests as thrush, which is the most common type of oropharyngeal candidiasis seen as creamy white exudative plaques on tongue, palate, tonsils and buccal mucosa. On removal of the white exudate raw bleeding buccal mucosa is observed (Fig. 6.10)

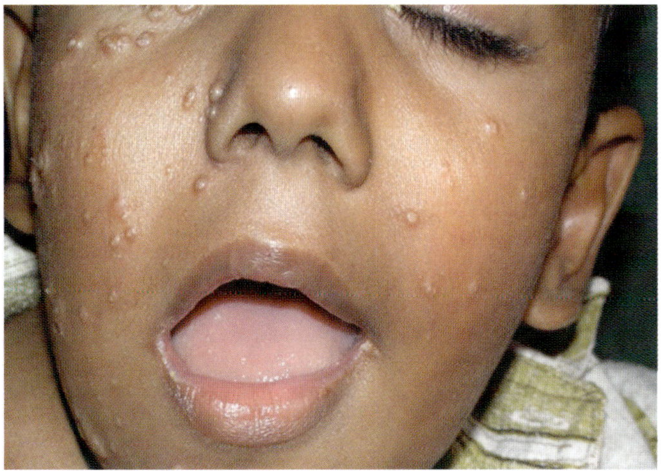

Fig. 6.5: Molluscum contagiosum on face with angular cheilitis

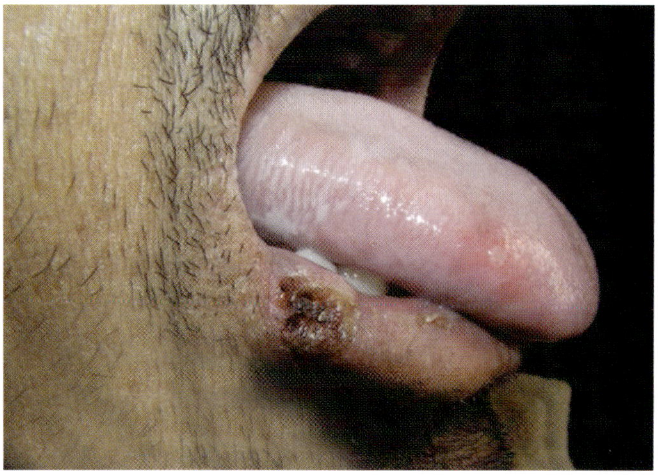

Fig.6.7: Oral hairy leukoplakia involving lateral border of tongue along with crusted lesion of herpes labialis

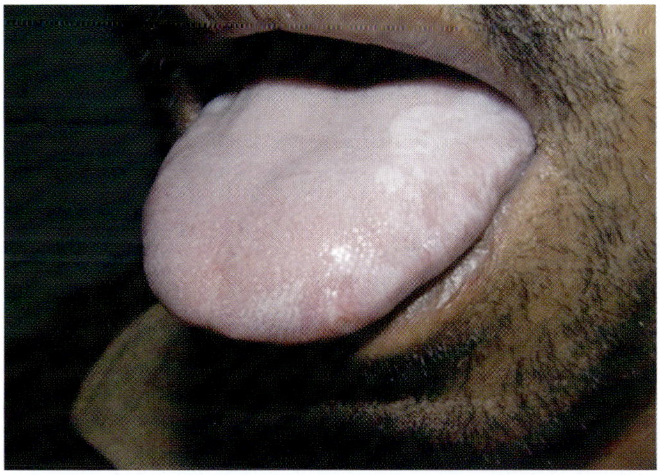

Fig. 6.6: Oral hairy leukoplakia over lateral border of tongue and lesion extending towards dorsum of tongue

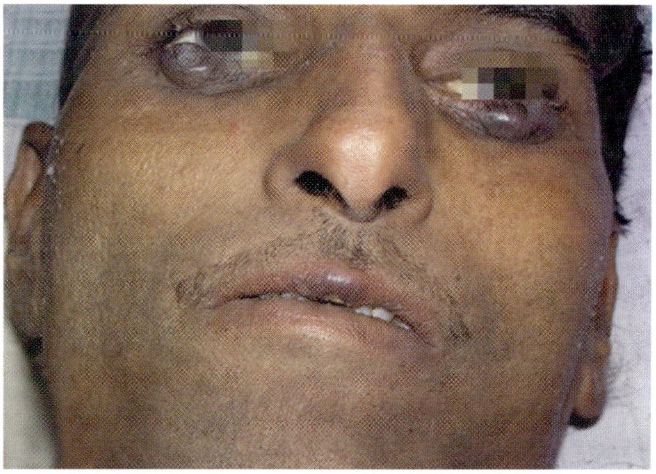

Fig. 6.8: Kaposi sarcoma on the upper lip

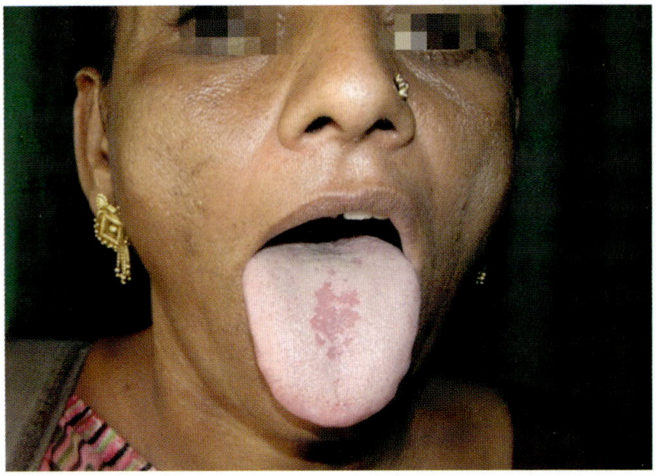

Fig. 6.9: Median rhomboid glossitis

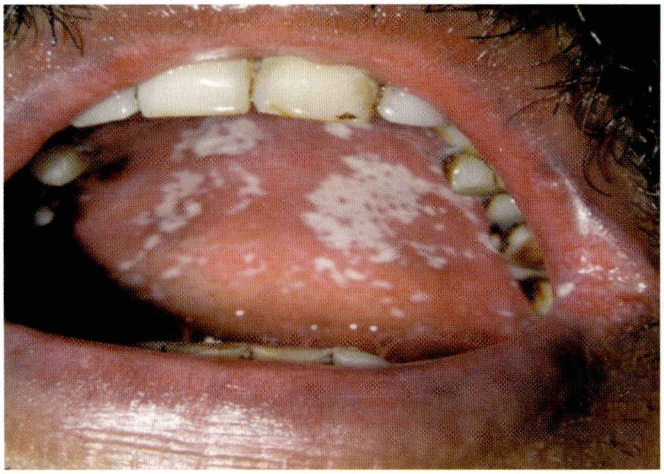

Fig. 6.10: Candidiasis on hard palate

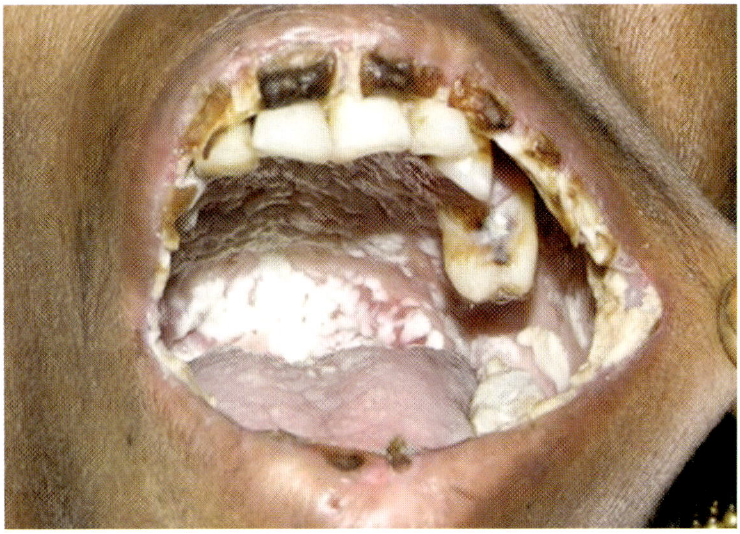

Fig. 6. 11: Extensire oral esophageal candidiasis and AIDS defining illness

- Other varieties of candidiasis are atrophic, hyperplastic, angular chelitis, median rhomboid glossitis, etc
- Esophageal candidiasis is the 2nd most common AIDS defining illness after *Pneumocystis Jirovecii* pneumonia (Fig. 6.11).

K. Cryptococcosis
- It is caused by *Paracoccidioides brasiliensis*. The condition clinically resembles actinomycosis, appearing as firm eroded or ulcerated swelling.

L. Mucocutaneous leishmaniasis
- It is caused by *Leishmania brasiliensis* and presents with lesions in oral cavity and lips as papule that ulcerates (Fig. 6.12)
- The ulcers are granulomatous and heal by fibrosis.

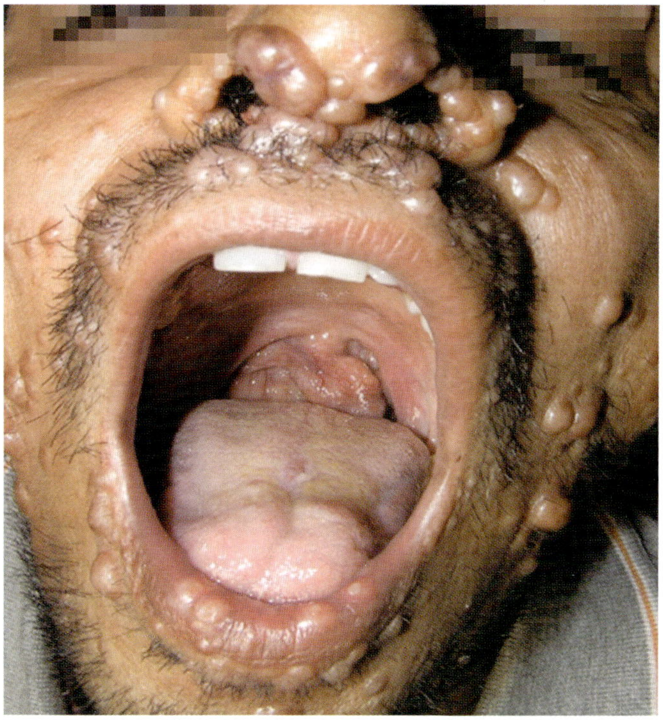

Fig. 6.12: Mucocutaneous leishmaniasis on lips and soft palate

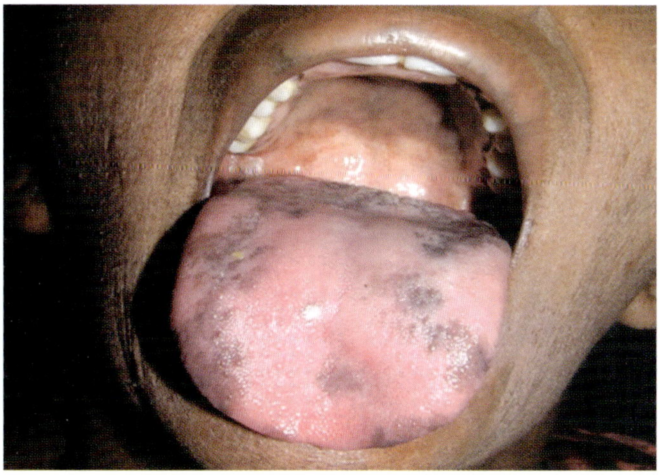

Fig. 6.13: Pigmentation over tongue

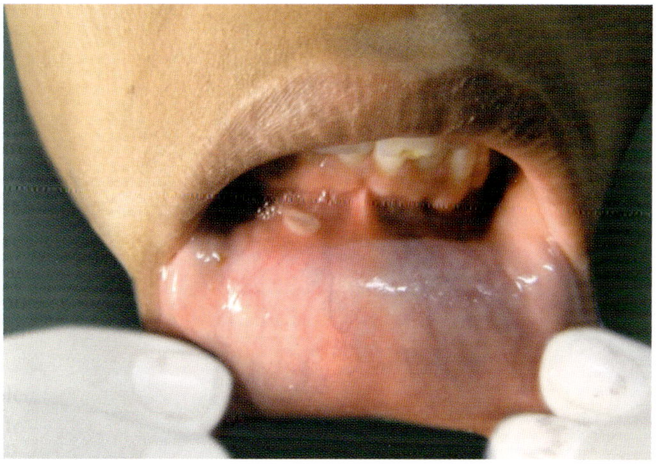

Fig. 6.14: Aphthous ulcer on lower lip

NONINFECTIOUS

A. Lichen planus
   - It can be an incidental finding in HIV patients
   - The most common presentation as reticular pattern others are plaque, atrophic, ulcerative or erosive, bullous variety
   - Oral LP is frequently associated with hepatitis C infection.

B. Recurrent aphthous stomatitis
   - It usually occurs in, otherwise, healthy individuals present as one or more painful recurrent ulcers on buccal (Fig. 6.14) and labial mucosa and tongue

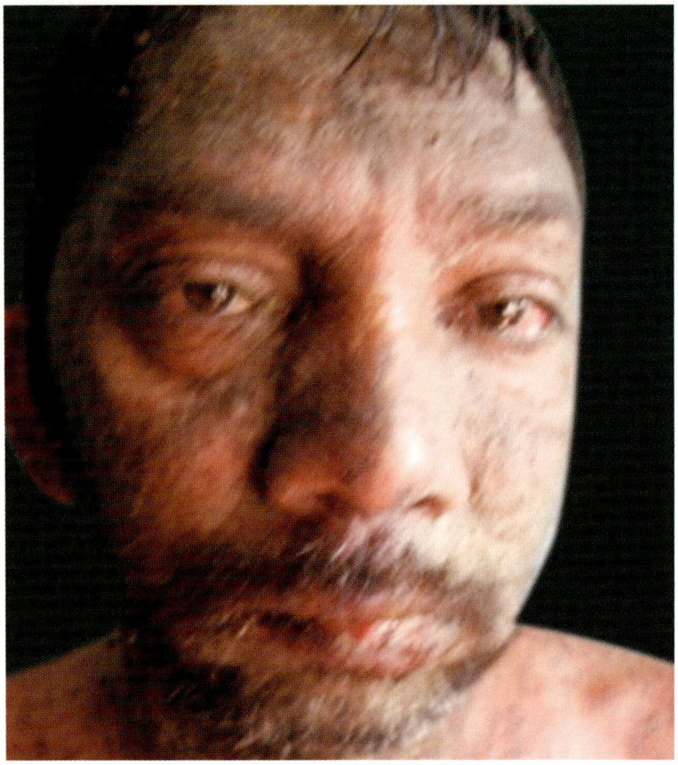

Fig. 6.15: Crusting and erosion on both lips due to SJ syndrome

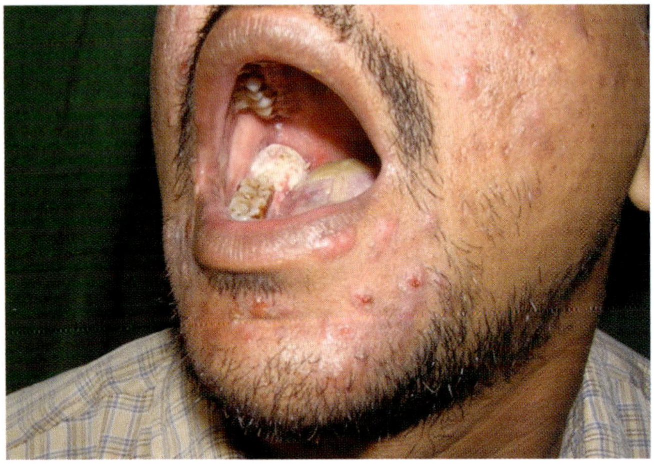

Fig. 6.16: Squamous cell carcinoma on buccal mucosa

- Increased CD8+:CD4+ T cell ratio, heredity, trauma, food, iron and B_{12} deficiency, stress, are possible etiologies
- Three type are known:
  1. Minor—3 mm to 1 cm
  2. Major—1 to 3 cm
  3. Herpetiform—extremely painful 1-3 mm size multiple pinpoint ulcers on any mucosat site may appear.

C. Reiter's disease
- Oral involvement is seen in 25% patients in general.
- Erythematous patches with superficial erosions on palate are characteristic findings.
- Tongue shows areas of erythema and loss of papillae.

D. Psoriasis
- Pustular psoriasis is associated with glossitis annular migrans geographic tongue.

E. Median Rhomboid Glossitis it is an oval or diamond shaped elevation seen over the dorsum of tongue more commonly in patients with suppressed immunity. (Fig. 6.9)

F. Pigmentation of oral cavity nonspecific pigmentation of oral cavity and tongue is very commonly encountered in HIV/AIDS patients (Fig. 6.13).

DRUG INDUCED

A. Steven Johnson syndrome
   - Cotrimoxazole and nevirapine are the most common culprits
   - Oral ulcers along with cutaneous lesions appear (Fig. 6.15).

MALIGNANCY

A. Leukoplakia
   - Presents as discrete, elevated, imbricated whitish plaque or patch that can not be rubbed off it has malignant potential
   - Surgical excision is indicated when cellular atypia is present.

B. Squamous cell carcinoma
   - May appear as exophytic or ulcerated growth. It may appear in the areas of leukoplakia (Fig. 6.16)
   - It is seen more commonly in tobacco chewer.

7 Dermatology in Cross-linked Hyaluronic Acid

HIV infection is becoming a prominent cause of childhood morbidity and mortality.

There is no single mucocutaneous disease that is pathognomonic in children with HIV infection.

Majority of these infection in HIV infected children can be distinguished from identical infection in healthy children only by the severity and frequency of recurrence (Figs 7.1 and 7.2).

CLINICAL SPECTRUM OF DERMATOLOGICAL MANIFESTATIONS

Infectious

Bacterial

- Impetigo and folliculitis may be recurrent and persistent in HIV disease, particularly in children. Most commonly caused by staphyloccocus and streptococcus (Figs 7.3 and 7.4)
- Disseminated furunculosis, gingivitis, gangrenous stomatitis and abscess formation can occur in patients with HIV infection
- Bacillary angiomatosis, which is caused by *Bartonella Hanselae* and rarely by *Bartonella quintana,* usually manifests as red papules and nodules
- Skin abscesses
- Ecthyma
- Cellulitis
- Mycobacterial infections (tuberculous and non-tuberculous) (Figs 7.5 and 7.6).

Viral Infections

Common viral infections in pediatric age group are:

- *Molluscum contagiosum*: MC lesions are small papules with central umbilication. In HIV infection, MC may be widespread and atypical. The lesions may be observed on unusual sites, such as the face, neck, and scalp, and the lesions may be of unusual morphology and size. Such unusual forms include solitary, endophytic, aggregated, inflamed and giant lesions (Figs 7.7 and 7.8)
- *Human papilloma virus*: Widespread or recalcitrant warts may be observed on the oral mucosa, the face, the perianal region, and the female genital tract in patients infected with HIV. Large plantar warts caused by HPV-66 and an epidermodysplasia

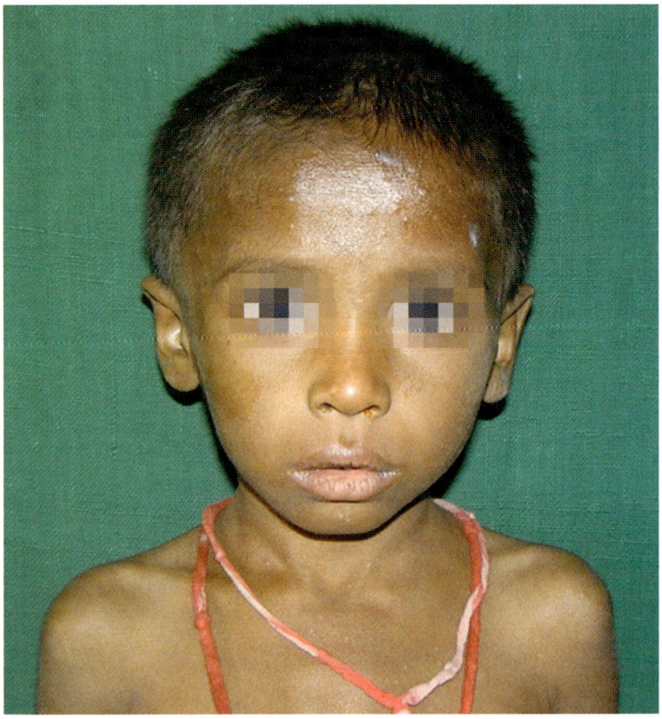

Fig. 7.1: Typical child living with HIV/AIDS

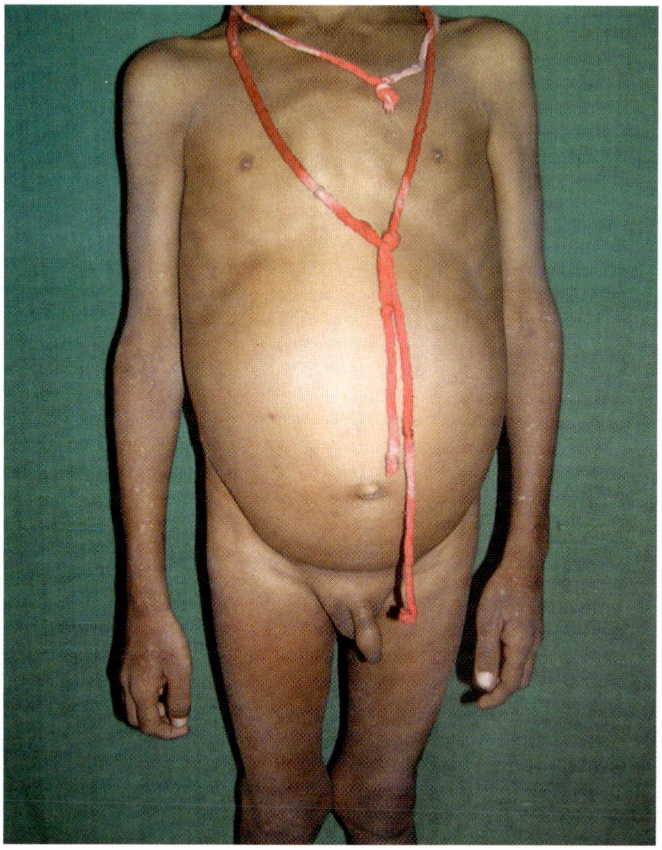

Fig.7.2: Pot belly

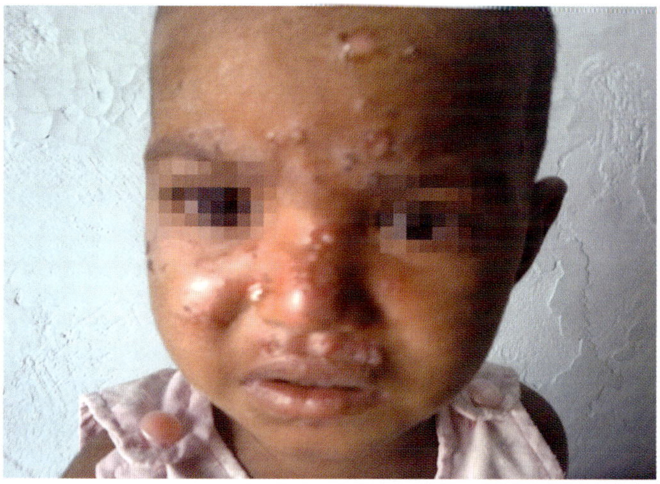

Fig. 7.3: Impetigo

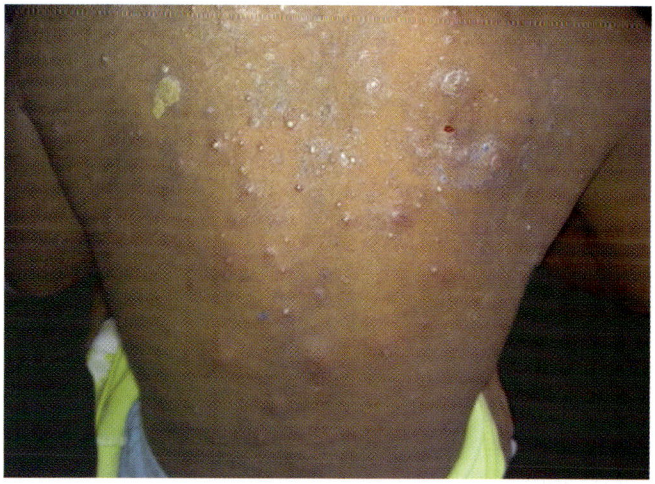

Fig. 7.4: Miliaria with periporitis

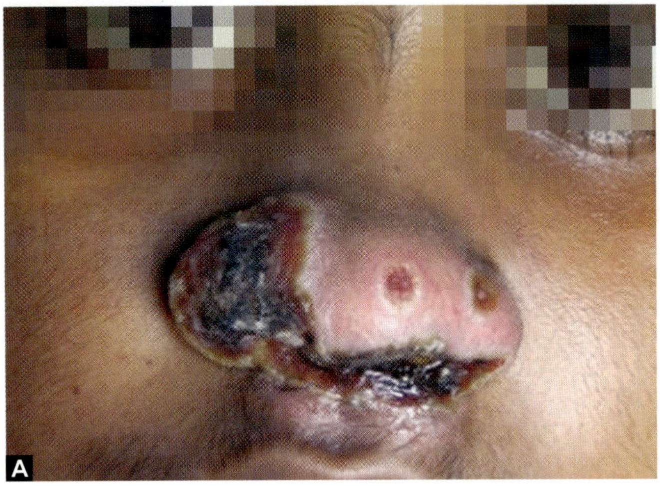

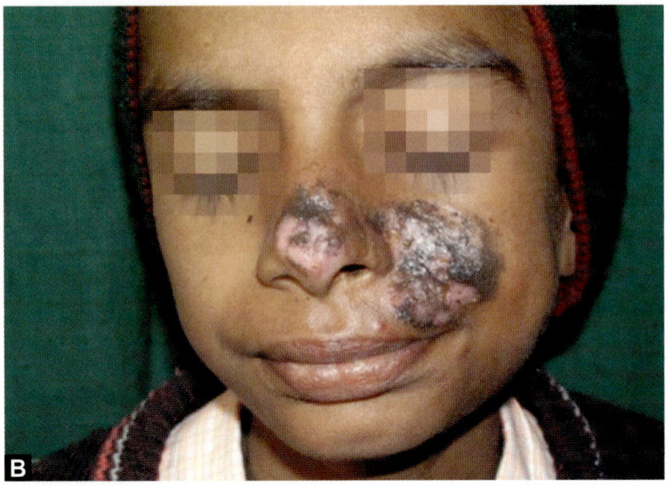

Figs 7.5A and B: Lupus vulgaris

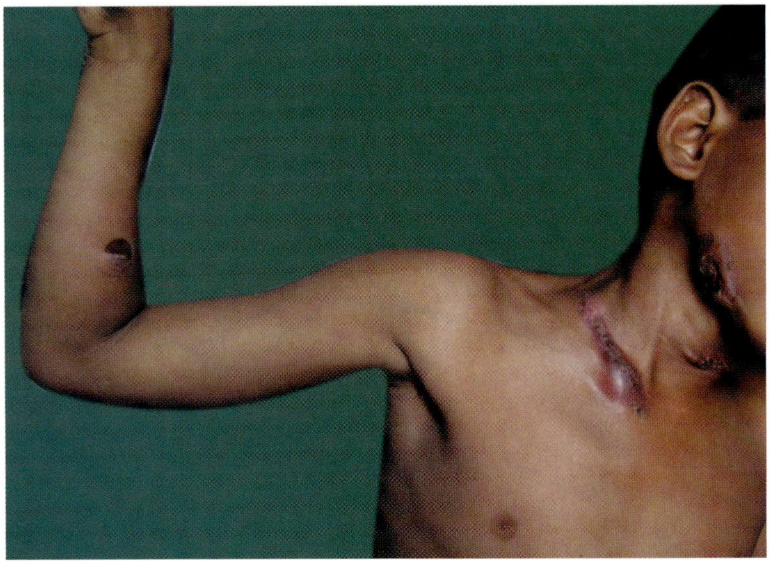

Fig. 7.6: Scrofuloderma at multiple sites with strong mantoux positivity

verruciformis like eruption, which is believed to be associated with HPV infection, have also been reported in patients infected with HIV (Fig. 7.9)

- Epstein-Barr virus (EBV) has been implicated in the pathogenesis of oral hairy leukoplakia. Oral hairy leukoplakia, which is characterized by filliform white serrations localized on the sides of the tongue, may develop in patients infected with HIV (Fig. 7.10)
- *Herpes simplex virus*: Gingivostomatitis, herpetic whitlow may be observed (Figs 7.11A and B)
- Measles
- Cytomegalovirus
- *Varicella-zoster virus*: Varicella, herpes zoster (Figs 7.12 to 7.15).

Fungal Infection

Superficial Fungal Infections

- Recurrent and persistent mucocutaneous candidiasis is common in patients with HIV infection

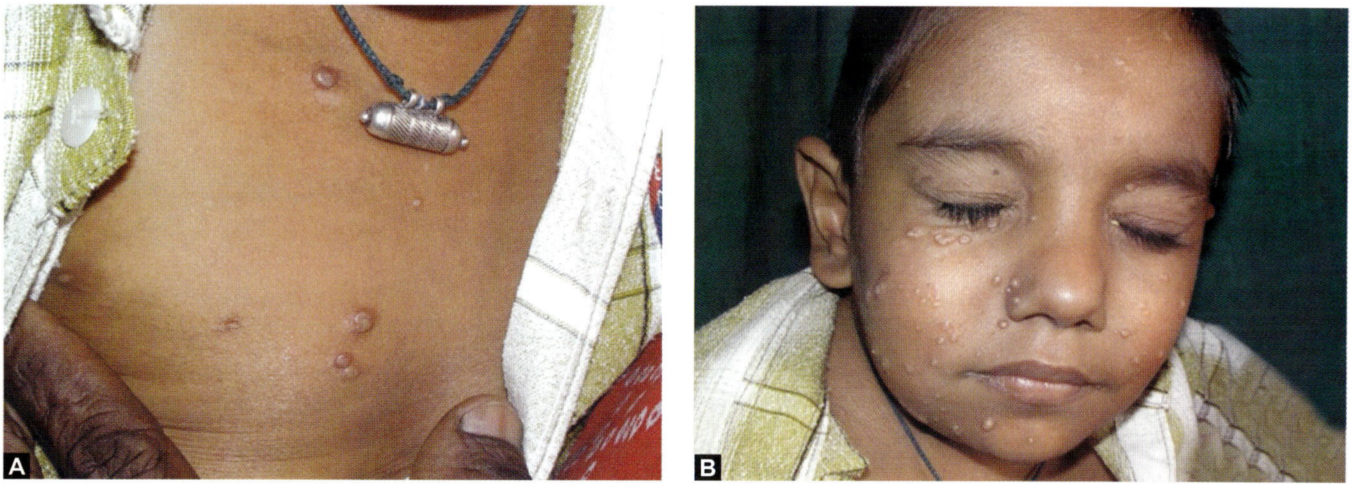

Figs 7.7A and B: Florid molluscum contagiosum over face and trunk

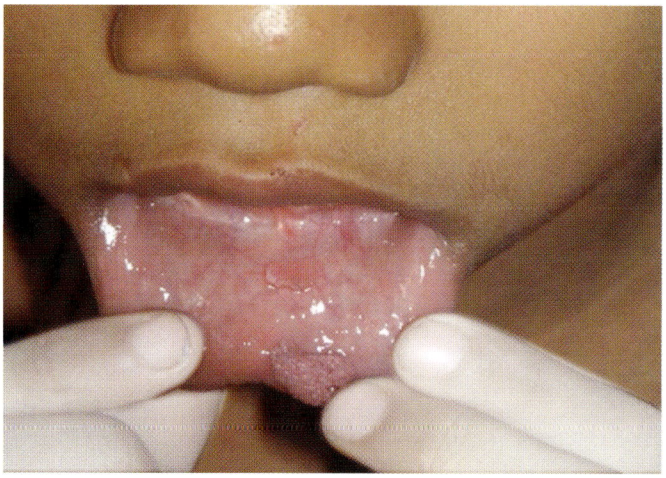

Fig. 7.8: Mucosal warts

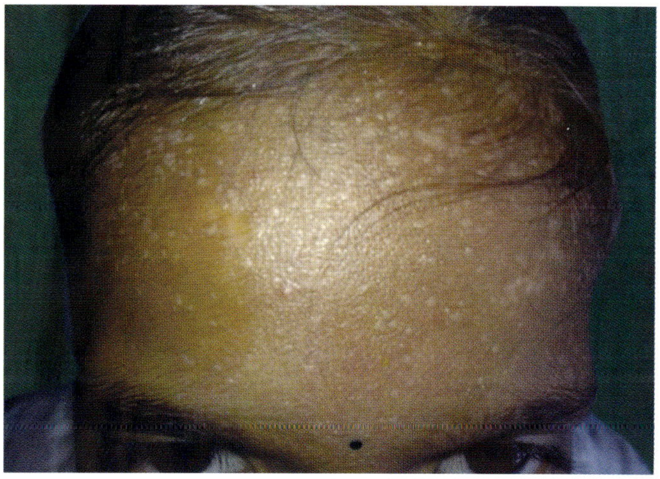

Fig. 7.9: Verruca plana

- Generalized dermatophytosis, or tinea capitis, which is typically caused by *Trichophyton rubrum*, may suggest HIV infection (Figs 7.16 to 7.19)
- Pityriasis versicolor may be persistent and recurrent in patients with HIV.

Deep Fungal Infections

- Rarely, cutaneous cryptococcosis may be observed in patients with HIV infection. Clinical manifestations include cellulitis; papules; plaques; ulcers; or translucent dome-shaped papules with central umbilication, resembling MC
- Cutaneous histoplasmosis presents as red papules, cellulitis like eruption, ulcerations, acneiform papules, or molluscum like lesions in patients infected with HIV
- North American blastomycosis may present as a disseminated maculopapular eruption in HIV disease

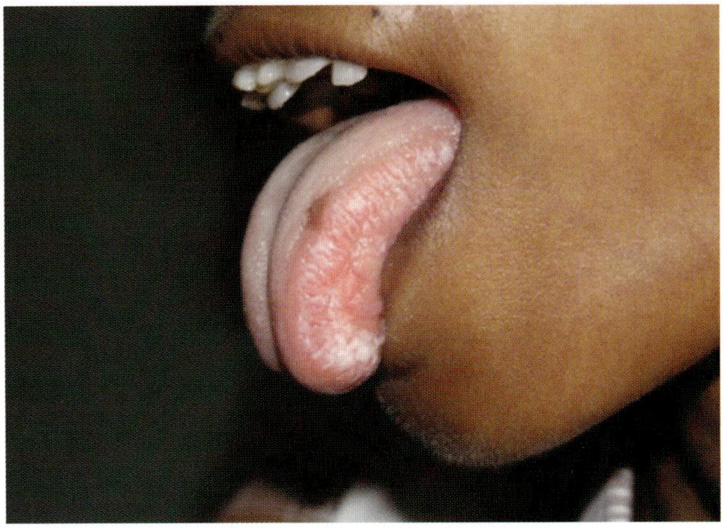

Fig. 7.10: Oral hairy leukoplakia

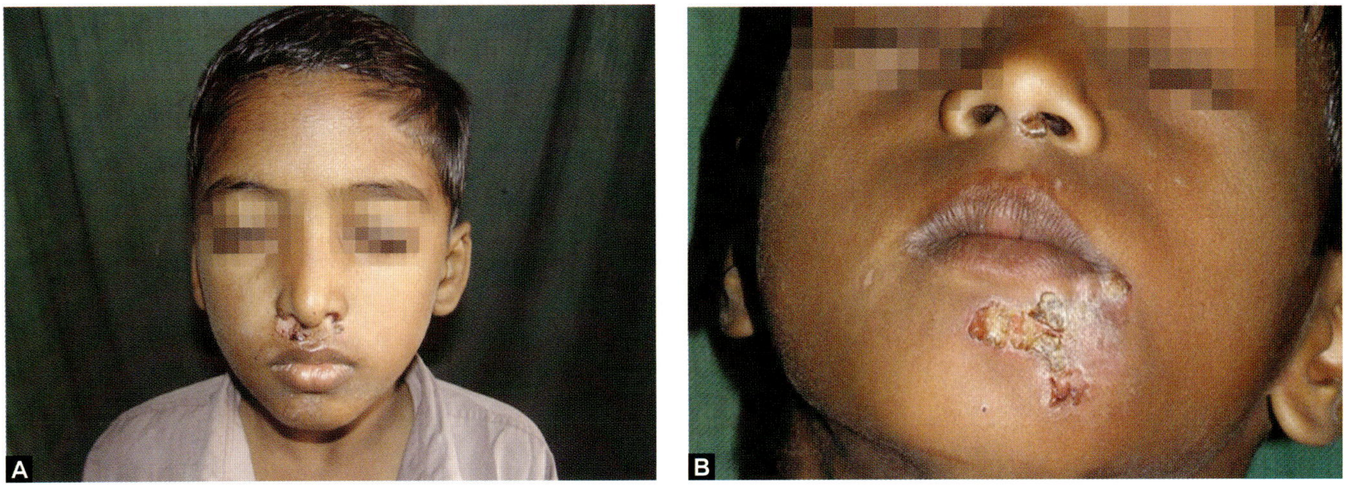

Figs 7.11A and B: Herpes labialis

- Systemic coccidioidomycosis may disseminate to the skin, usually as hemorrhagic papules or nodules.

Infestations

- *Scabies*: Atypical or Norwegian scabies, which is characterized by widespread hyperkeratotic, scaly maculopapular eruptions or crusted plaques, can occur in patients with HIV infection
- *Demodicidosis*: *Demodex folliculorum* folliculitis may lead to a pruritic papular eruption (PPE) on the face and the upper part of the trunk in patients with HIV disease
- Pediculosis.

Noninfectious (Inflammatory Dermatoses)

- Generalized dry skin syndrome is frequently observed in patients with HIV infection. Xerosis may

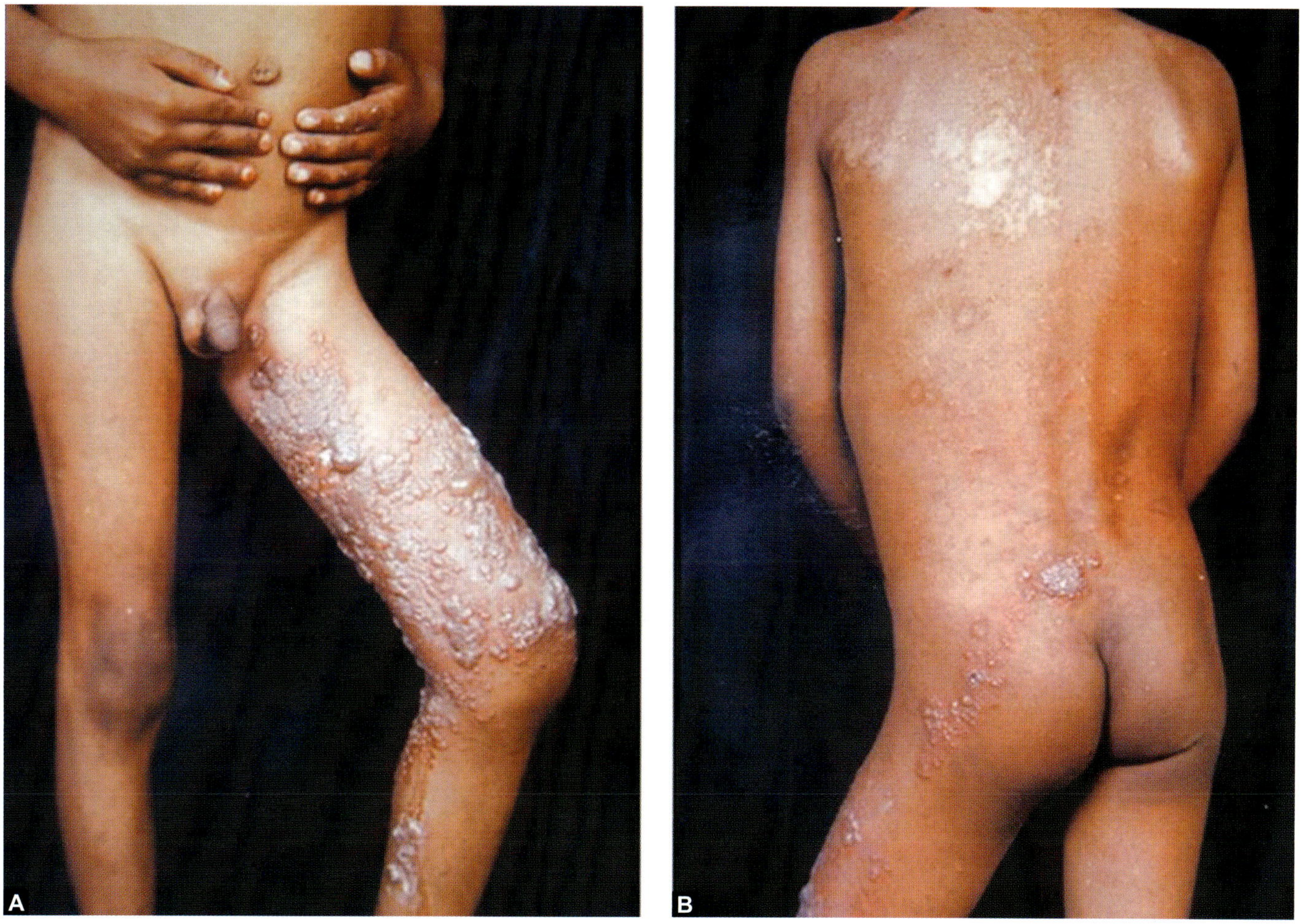

Figs 7.12A and B: Multidermatomal herpes zoster with previous scars in thoracic dermatomes

be the initial clinical manifestation of AIDS and is often a cause of pruritus (Figs 7.20A and B).

- *Seborrheic dermatitis*: Seborrheic dermatitis may be the initial cutaneous manifestation of HIV disease. The eruption, which is characterized by widespread inflammatory and hyperkeratotic lesions, may progress to erythroderma in some patients (Fig. 7.21)
- *Pruritic papular eruption*: PPE is a common cutaneous manifestation in patients infected with HIV. It manifests as small, itchy, red or skin-colored papules over the head, neck and upper part of body (Figs 7.22A to C).
- Eosinophilic folliculitis manifests as an idiopathic, highly pruritic, papulopustular eruption of sterile pustules involving the face, neck, trunk, and extremities
- Urticaria
- Psoriasis (Figs 7.23A and B)
- Acquired ichthyosis may begin on the lower extremities and disseminate in advanced HIV disease. Acquired ichthyosis may be a marker of concomitant infection with HIV-1 and human lymphotropic virus II in persons who use intravenous drugs and have profound helper T cell depletion.
- Aphthous ulcers
- Pyoderma gangrenosum
- Sweet syndrome
- Eosinophilic vasculitis.

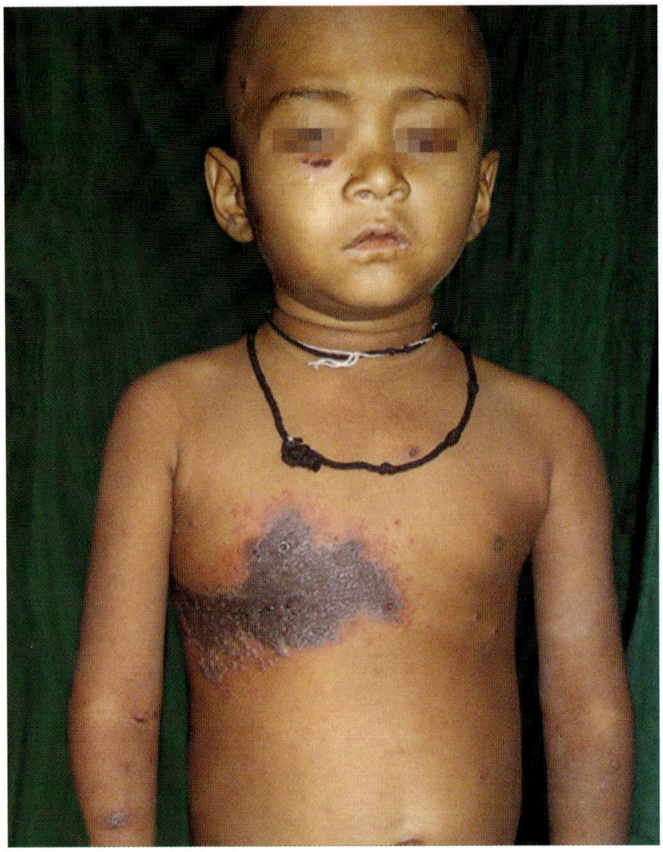

Fig. 7.13: Hemorrhagic herpes zoster

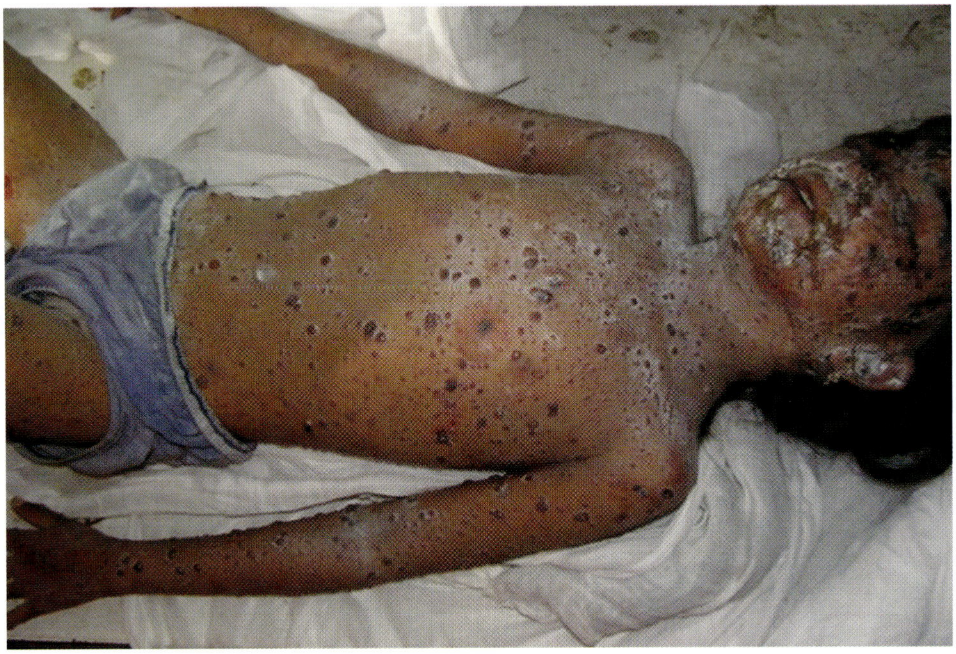

Fig. 7.14: Hemmorhagic varicella with encephalitis

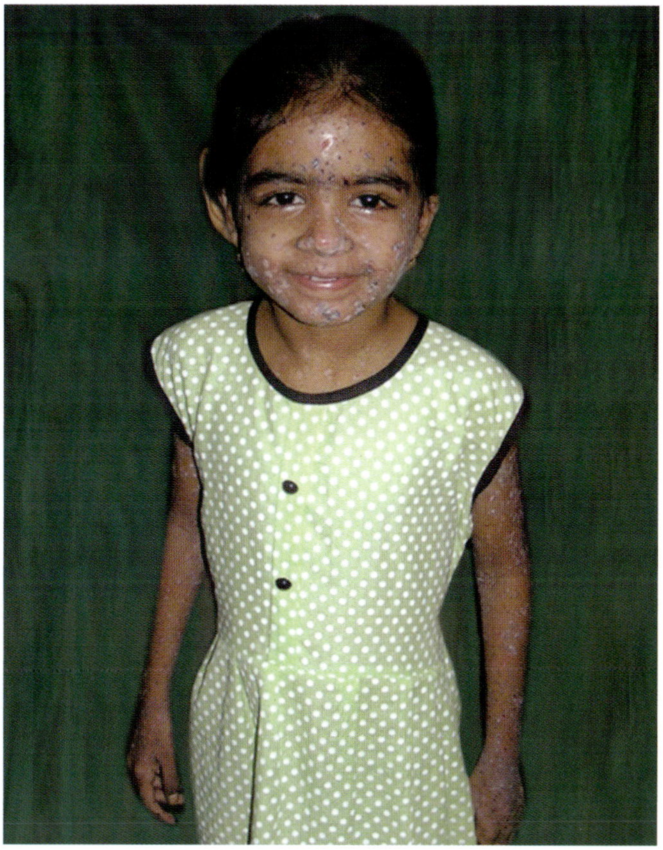

Fig. 7.15: Follow-up after IV acyclovir therapy for 7 days

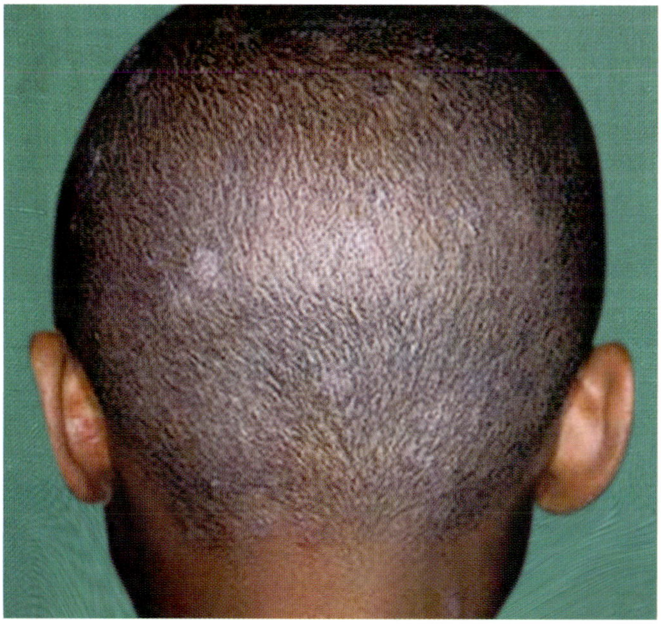

Fig. 7.16: T. capitis with T. corporis

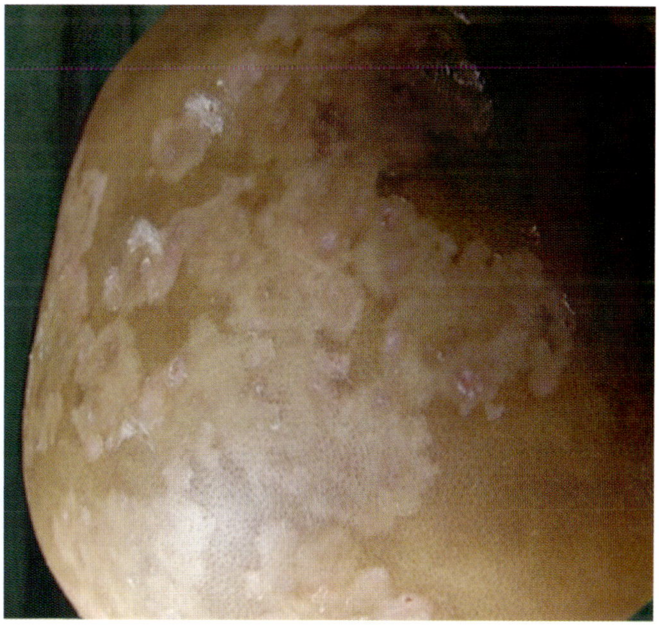

Fig. 7.17: Tinea capitis

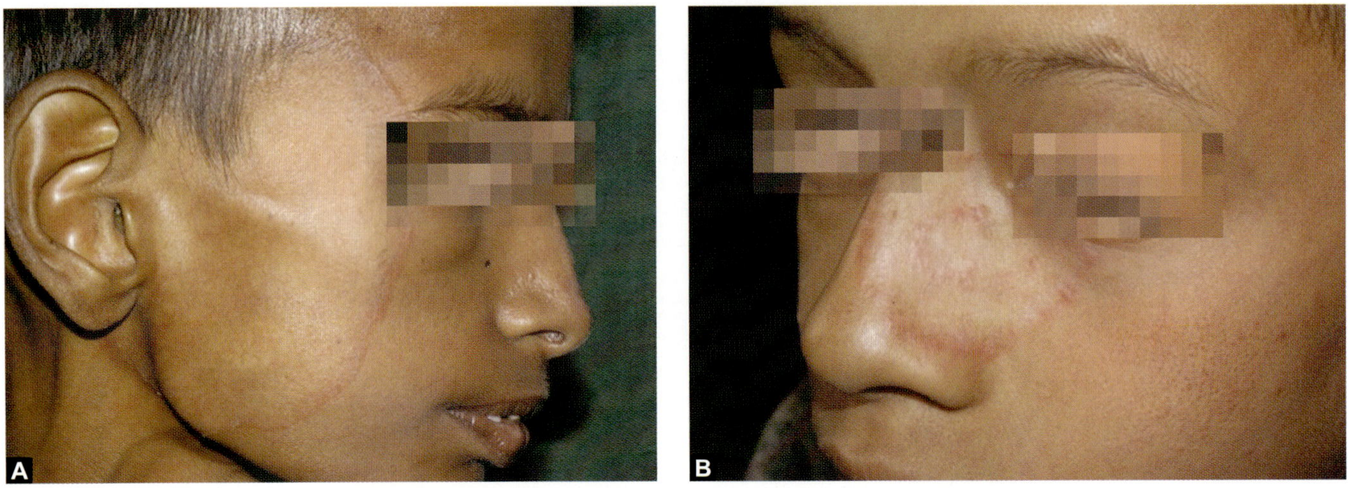

Figs 7.18A and B: Tinea faciei

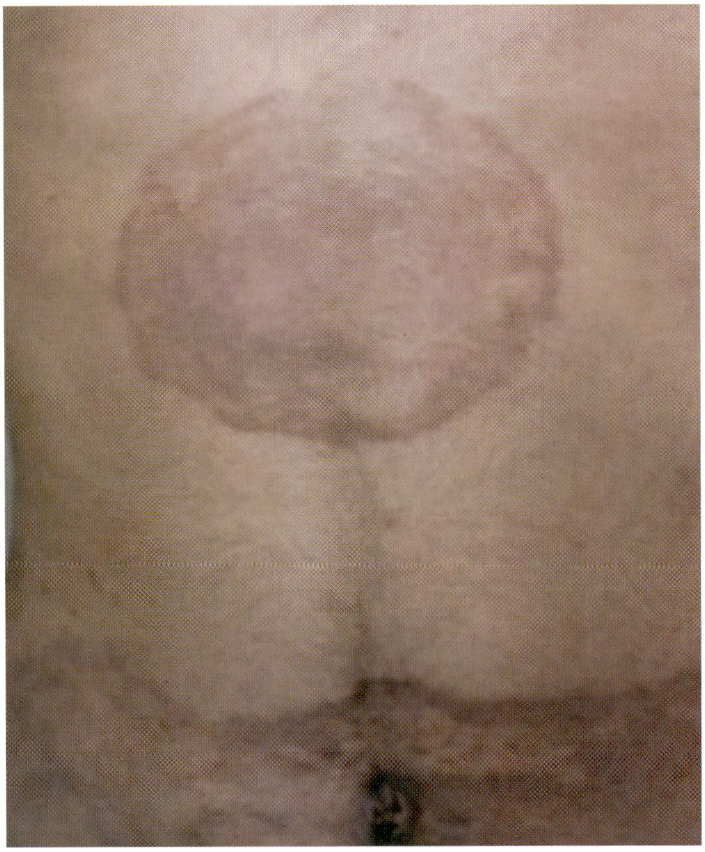

Fig. 7.19: Tinea imbricata

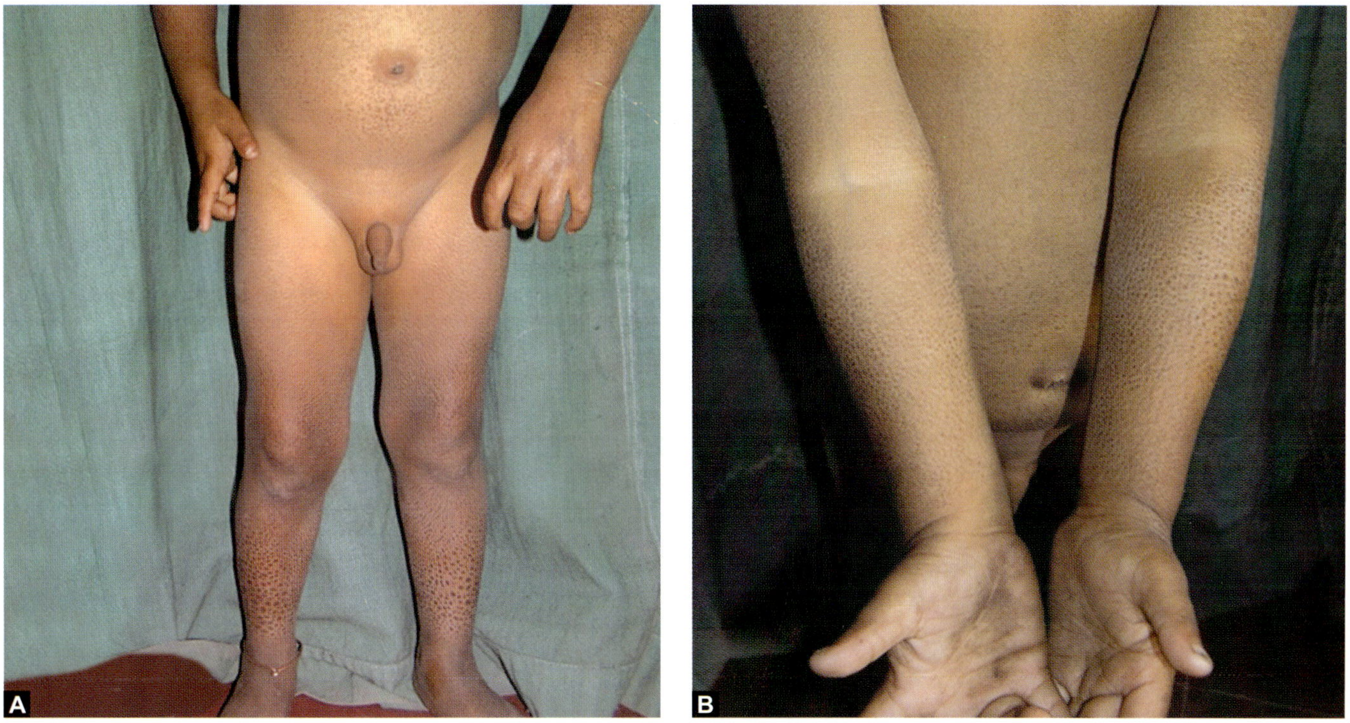

Figs 7.20A and B: Severe xerosis in a dermatology in cross-linked hyaluronic acid (CLHA)

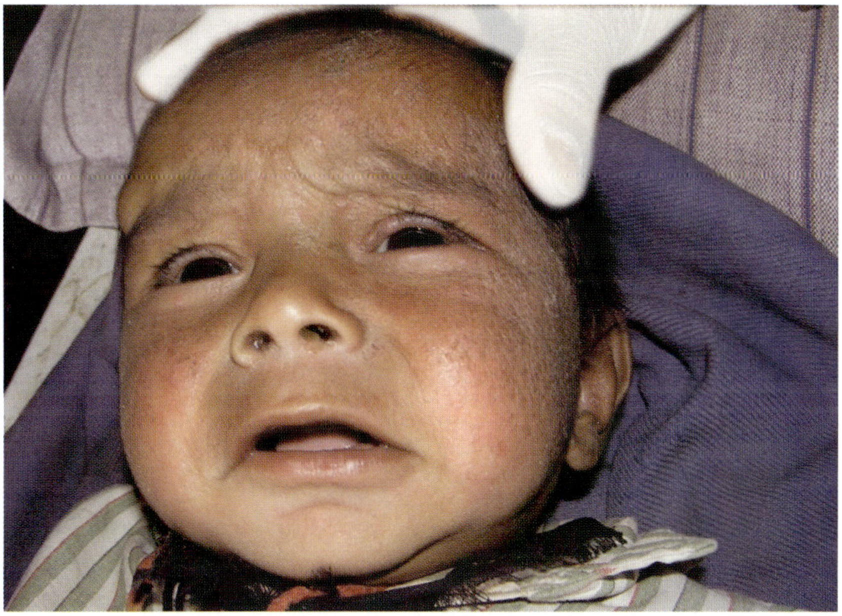

Fig. 7.21: Seborrheic dermatitis on the face

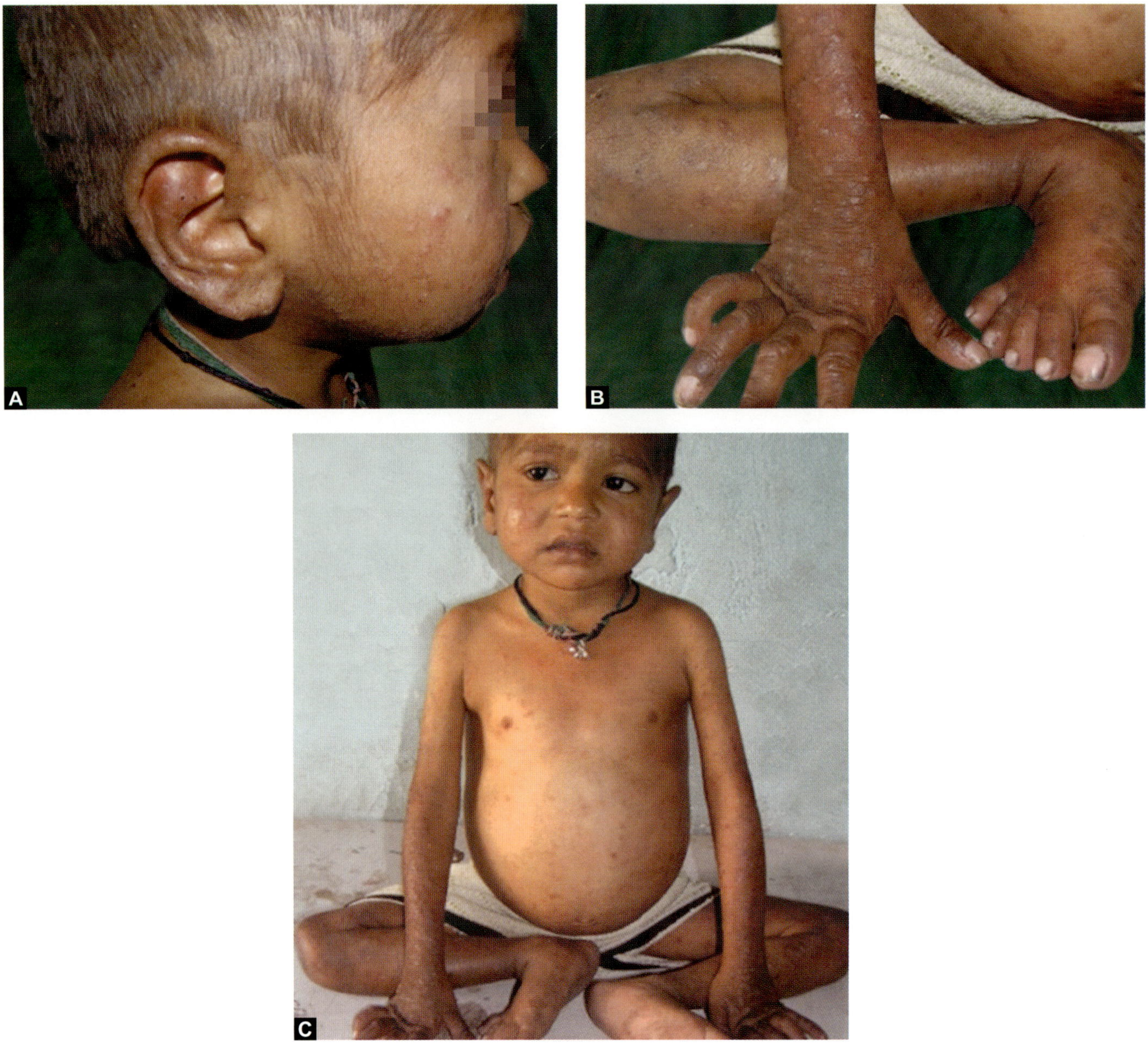

Figs 7.22A to C: Prupritic popular eruptions over face and extremities

Hair and Nail Disorders

- Diffuse alopecia or alopecia areata may be associated with HIV disease and may be inflammatory and permanent. The apoptotic follicular stem cell population in higher proportion may represent a hair cycle disturbance in patients with diffuse alopecia related to HIV-1 infection
- Generalized alopecia can occur in patients with HIV who are treated with indinavir, an antiretroviral protease inhibitor

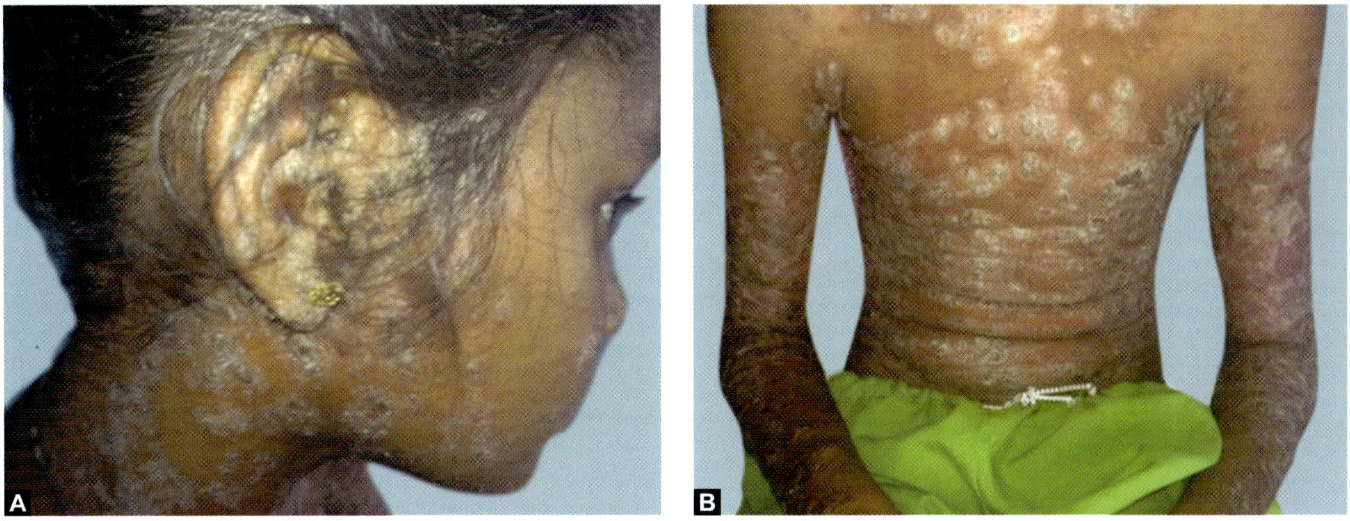

Figs 7.23A and B: Psoriasis

- Elongation of the eyelashes and softening and straightening of the scalp hair may be observed in HIV disease
- Beau's lines, telogen effluvium, and pallor of the nail beds are the general effects of the chronic illness
- Zidovudine is associated with longitudinal, transverse, or diffuse melanin pigmentation of the nails; however, nail pigmentation has also been observed in patients with HIV who have never received zidovudine
- Proximal white onychomycosis is usually a sign of HIV disease.

8 Immune Reconstitution Inflammatory Syndrome

DEFINITION

- *Synonyms*: Immune restoration disease
- Immune reconstitution inflammatory syndrome (IRIS) or immune reconstitution syndrome (IRS) is a condition seen in some cases of AIDS in which the immune system begins to recover, but then responds to a previously acquired opportunistic infection with an overwhelming inflammatory response that paradoxically makes the symptoms of infection worse
- To diagnose or define above condition, close observation by the clinician is needed when starting Highly active antiretroviral therapy (HAART) on HIV/AIDS patients with known history of opportunistic infection
- Because definition of IRIS is one of clinical suspicion and disease specific criteria yet to be developed, determining true incidence is difficult.

PATHOGENESIS OF IRIS

- Despite numerous descriptions of the manifestations of IRIS, its pathogenesis remains largely specculative
- Combination of
  - Underlying antigen burden
  - Degree of immune restoration host genetic susceptibility
- These pathogenic mechanisms may interact and are likely to depend on the underlying burden of infectious or noninfectious agent.

Antigenic Burden

- Whether elicited by an infectious or noninfectious agent, the presence of an antigenic stimulus for development of the syndrome appears necessary
- This antigenic stimulus can be intact, 'clinically silent' organisms or dead or dying organisms and their residual antigens
- IRIS that occurs as a result of 'unmasking' of clinically silent infection is characterized by atypical exuberant inflammation and/or an accelerated clinical presentation suggesting a restoration of antigen-specific immunity. These characteristics differentiate IRIS from incident opportunistic infections that occur on ART as a result of delayed adequate immunity.

DEGREE OF IMMUNE RESTORATION FOLLOWING HAART

- The suppression of CD4 T cells by HIV causes a decrease in the body's normal response to certain infections. Not only this there is more difficulty to fight the infection, it may mean that a level of infection that would normally produce symptoms is instead undetected (subclinical infection)
- If the CD4 count rapidly increases (due to effective treatment of HIV, or removal of other causes of immunosuppression), a sudden increase in the inflammatory response produces nonspecific symptoms such as fever and in some cases a worsening of damage to the infected tissue.

Other Factors

- Enhanced pathogen specific immunity
- HAART shifts balance from Th-2 to Th-1 cytokine response resulting in exacerbation of pro-inflammatory cytokines.

RISK FACTORS FOR DEVELOPMENT OF IRIS

- Male sex
- Younger age
- Lower CD4 cell count at ART initiation
- Higher HIV RNA at ART initiation
- Lower CD4 cell percentage at ART initiation
- *Lower CD4*:CD8 ratio at ART initiation
- More rapid initial fall in HIV RNA on ART
- Antiretroviral *naïve* at time of OI diagnosis
- Shorter interval between OI therapy initiation and ART initiation.

TYPES OF IRIS

1. '*Unmasking Iris*': The first is the 'unmasking' of an occult opportunistic infection. In unmasking IRIS, the most common treatment is to administer an antibiotic or antiviral drugs against the infectious organism. In some severe cases, anti-inflammatory medications, such as corticosteroids are needed to suppress inflammation until the infection has been eliminated.
2. '*Paradoxical Iris*': The second is the 'paradoxical' symptomatic relapse of a prior infection despite microbiologic treatment success. Often in paradoxical IRIS, microbiologic cultures are sterile. In paradoxical IRIS reactions, the events will usually spontaneously get better with time without any additional therapy.

Clinical Spectrum of IRIS

Bacterial Infections

- *Mycobacterium tuberculosis (Figs 8.3 to 8.5)*
- *Mycobacterium avium* complex
- *Pneumocystis jivoreci*/PCP
- *Mycobacterium leprae* (Borderline tuberculoid)
- *Bartonella henselae.*

Viral Infections

- Herpes simplex virus
- Vericella-zoster virus (Fig. 8.1)
- Molluscum contagiosum virus (Fig. 8.2)
- Cytomegalovirus
- Epstein-Barr virus

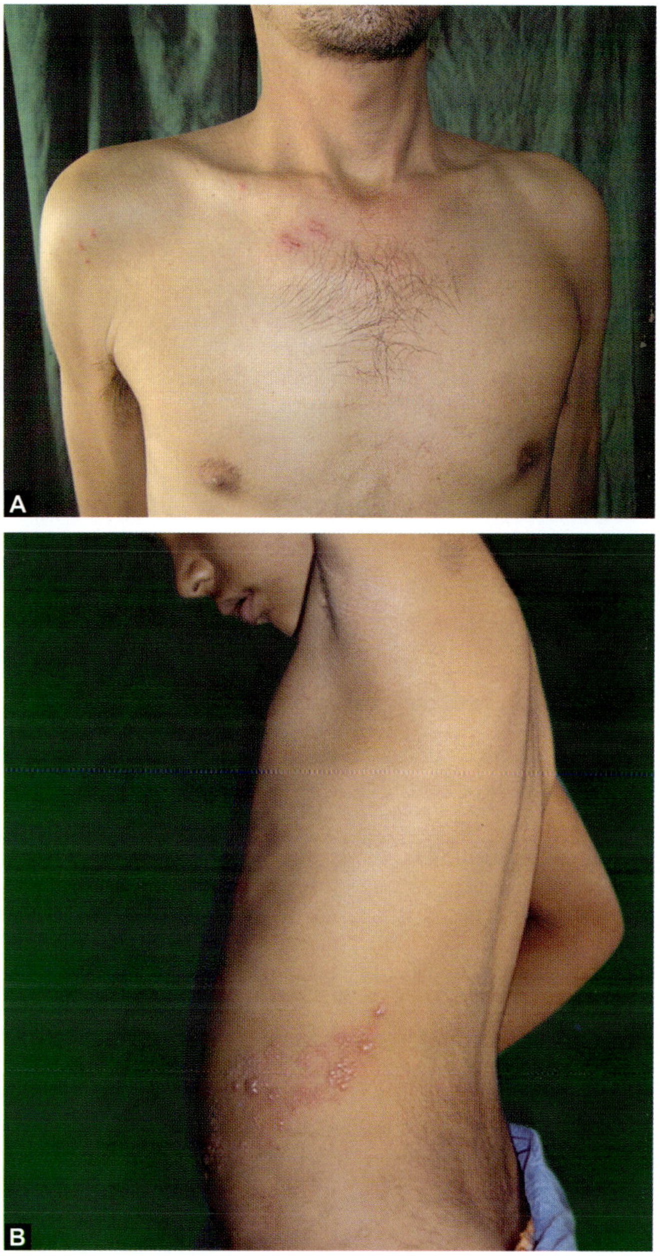

Figs 8.1A and B: Herpes zoster as IRIS in adult and child

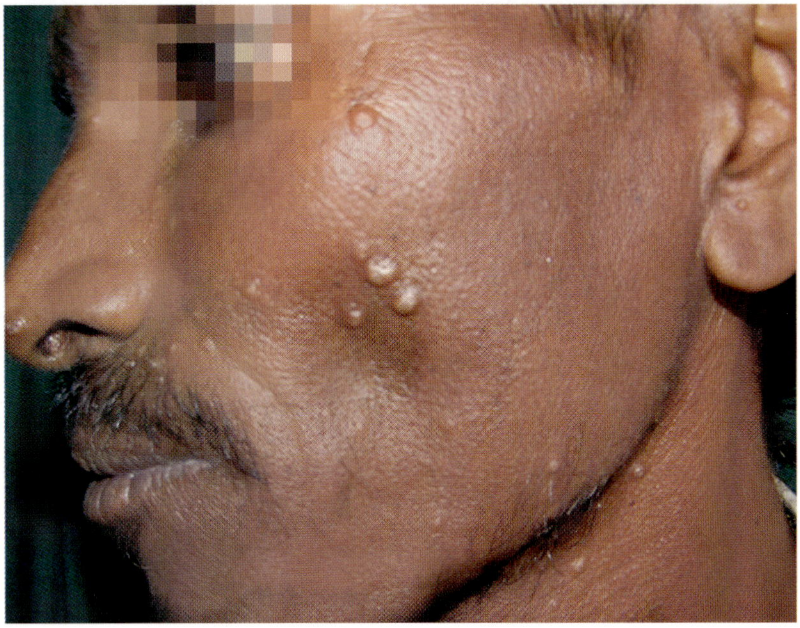

Fig. 8.2: Molluscum presenting as IRIS

- HHV-8 (Castleman's/Kaposi)
- Hepatitis B and C virus
- Human papilloma virus
- JC virus (PML).

Fungal and Protozoal Infections

- *Cryptococcus neoformans*
- *Histoplasma capsulatum*
- *Toxoplasma gondii*
- Microsporodioses
- Leishmaniasis.

Autoimmune Conditions

- Grave's disease
- Sarcoidosis
- Systemic lupus erythematosus
- Rheumatoid arthritis
- Polymyositis
- Guillian-Barre syndrome
- Alopecia universalis
- Vasculitis.

Gastrointestinal Inflammation

- Appendicitis
- Cholecystitis
- Splenitis.

Dermatosis

- Eosinophilic folliculitis
- Hyperallergic/allergic reactions.

Proposed Criteria for Diagnosing IRIS

- The patient has to be on ART with a rising CD4 cell count and falling viral load
- Prior to starting ART, the patient has to had a clinical response to treatment of one of the three opportunistic infections listed above

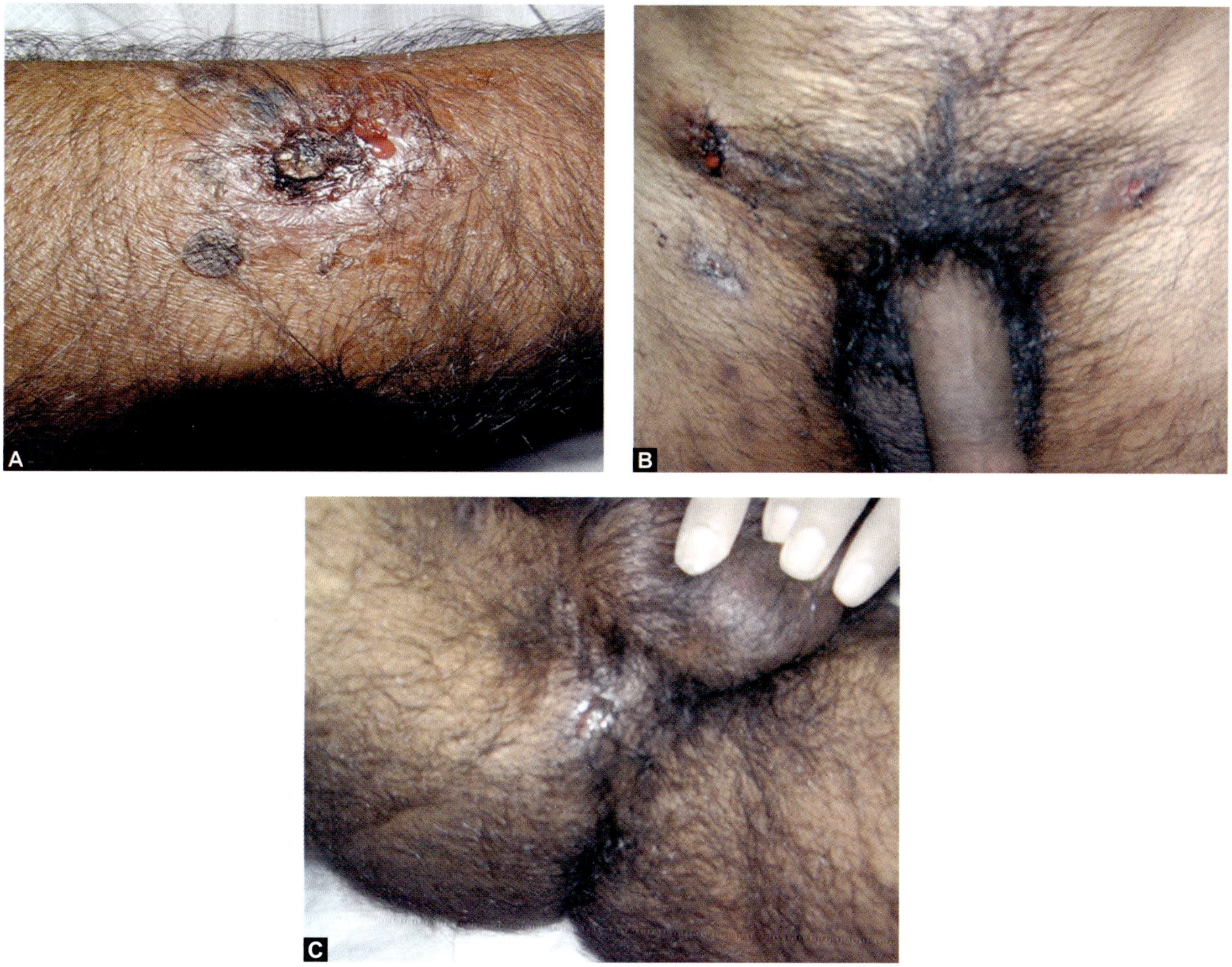

Figs 8.3A to C: Scrofuloderma at 3 sites—as IRIS

- Following the initiation of ART, the patient has to have either recurrence of their initial symptoms or new symptoms of an inflammatory process that is not consistent with the usual course of an established infection or a new infection
- All cultures or other lab studies carried out because of the OI 'flare-up' has to be negative (in other words, lab studies needed to show that the infection process itself is not spreading or worsening).

Criteria by French et al, 2004

Major Criteria

- Atypical presentation of OI or tumor in patient on HAART
- Exaggerated inflammatory response like fever, painful lesions
- Atypical inflammatory response in affected tissues like granuloma, suppuration or necrosis

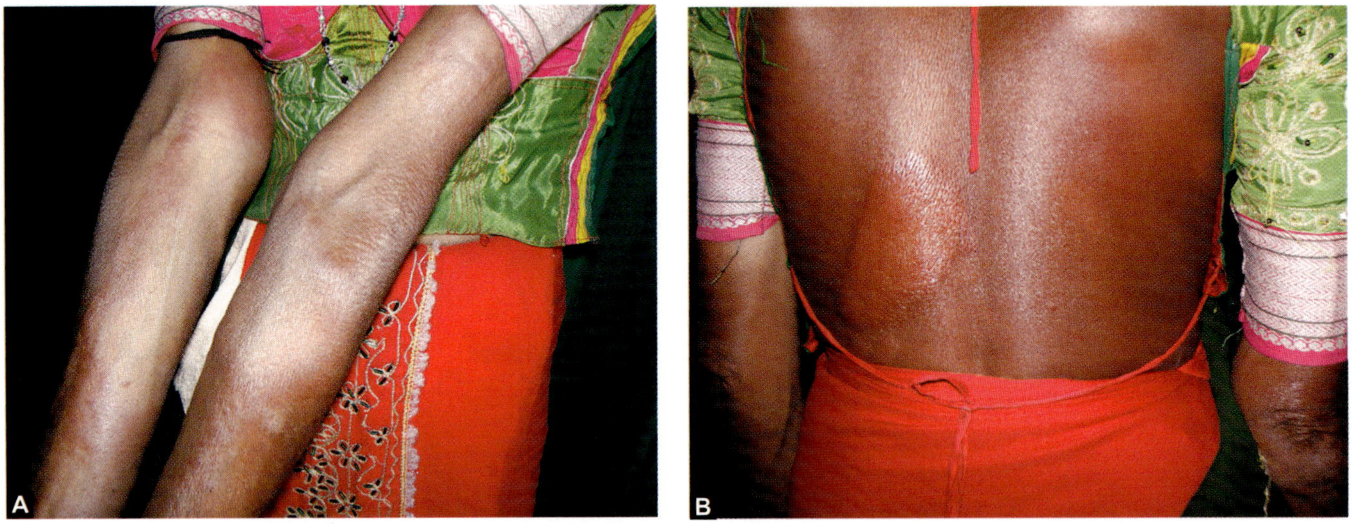

Figs 8.4A and B: Borderline tuberculoid Hansen's in a female presenting as IRIS

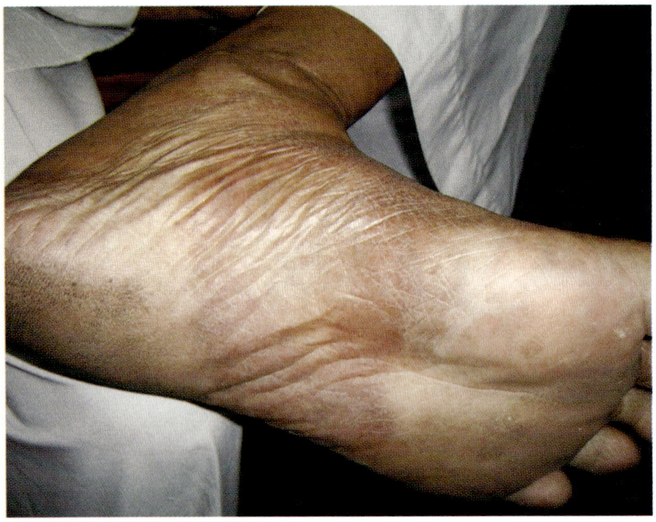

Fig. 8.5: Tuberculoid leprosy as IRIS

- Progression of organ dysfunction or enlargement of pre-existing lesions after definite clinical improvement with specific OI therapy and exclusion of toxicity prior to starting HAART like tuberculosis, worsening Kaposi's, new onset CMV retinitis or CMV uveitis
- Reduction in plasma HIV RNA by > 1 log 10 copies per ml.

Minor Criteria

- Increase in CD4 count
- Increase in specific immune response to pathogen
- Spontaneous resolution of disease without specific therapy with continuing antiretroviral therapy.

9 Drug Reactions

WHO defines ADR: "A response to a drug that is noxious and unintended and occurs at doses normally used in man for prophylaxis to diagnoses or therapy of disease, or for the modification of physiological function."

CLASSIFICATION OF ADR

Type A (Augmented)

- These reactions are dose related and include toxic effects and side effects.

Type B (Bizarre)

- Reactions are neither dose related nor related to pharmacology
- They include immunological hypersensitivity and idiosyncratic reactions such as Steven Johnson syndrome (SJS), toxic epidermal necrolysis (TEN), drug hypersensitivity syndrome (DHS).

Type C (Chronic)

- These reactions are related to cumulative dose and time.

Type D (Delayed)

- These reactions are time-related, becoming apparent sometime after the use of drug.

Type E (Withdrawal)

- Reactions occur at the end of use.

Type F (Failure)

- These reactions occur as a consequence of drug interactions and leading to failure of therapy and are thus dose related
- Adverse drug reactions manifesting in the skin and mucous membrane are a common finding in HIV/AIDS, are attributable to antimicrobial agents and/or antiretroviral agents.

CHALLENGES TO ANTIBACTERIAL AND ANTIRETROVIRAL THERAPY IN HIV

- The potential for adverse drug reaction influences the choice of medications and patient's ability to continue treatment
- The risk for these ADR is greatly increased due to the underlying immune dysfunction and the fact that multiple drugs are often prescribed simultaneously.

Reported side effects are as follows:

1. *Morbilliform rash*: Exanthematous eruptions probably account for the vast majority of drug induced skin rashes. The combination of trimethoprim and sulfamethoxazole, commonly administered for prophylaxis against *Pneumocystis jirovecii* pneumonia, is notoriously responsible for this reaction. Other sulfonamides and penicillins may also trigger this reaction (Fig. 9.1).
2. *Urticaria*: It consists of raised, erythmatous skin lesions that are markedly pruritic, evanescent and generally worsened by scratching (Fig. 9.2).
3. *Angioedema*: It is a reaction similar to urticaria except that massive edema involves the

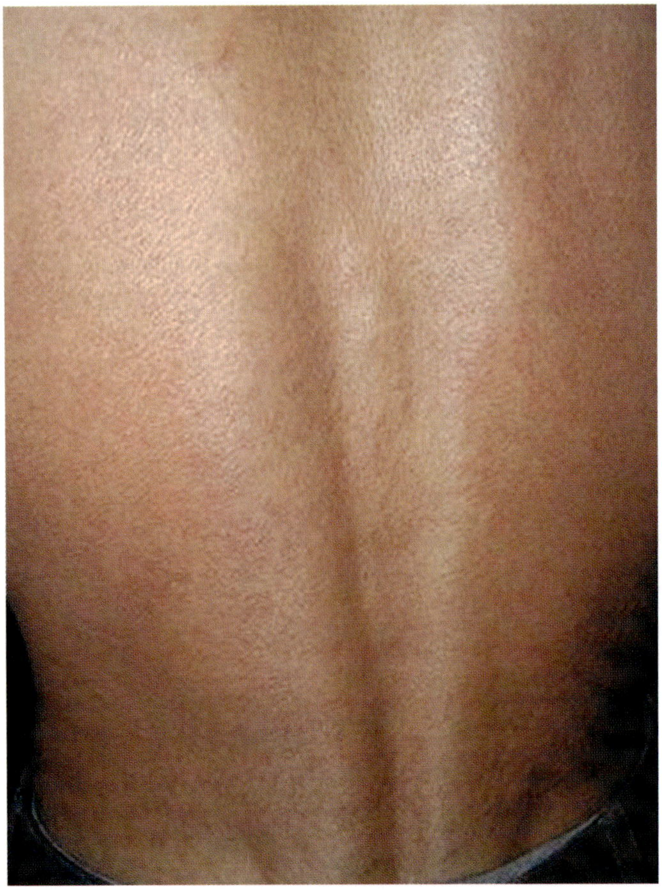

Fig. 9.1: Morbilliform rash

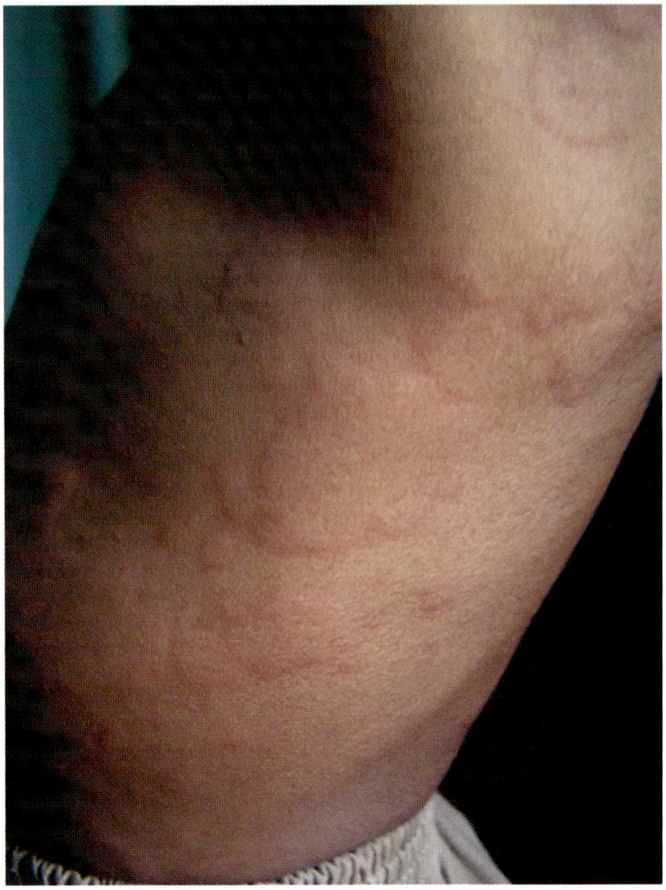

Fig. 9.2: Acute urticaria

subcutaneous tissues rather than the dermis. It is clinically characterized by asymmetric swelling of tissues with overlying normal looking skin and by patients having more burning than itching (Fig. 9.3).

4. *Fixed drug eruption*: Fixed drug eruptions (FDEs) characteristically recur in the same site or sites each time a particular drug is taken; with each exposure however, the number of involved sites may increase (Fig. 9.4).
5. *Erythema multiforme*: Clinically, macular, papular or urticarial lesions, as well as classical iris or target lesions; are distributed preferentially on the distal extremities. Lesions may involve palm, trunk as well as genital mucous membrane. Neviapine, abacavir and trimethoprim-sulfamethoxazole may commonly trigger these lesions (Figs 9.5 and 9.6).
6. *Steven Johnson syndrome*: It is a severe illness of sudden onset, associated with marked constitutional symptoms of high fever, malaise, myalgia, arthralgia, and extensive EM of the trunk, with occasional skin blisters and erosions covering less than 10% of the body surface area (Figs 9.7 to 9.9).
7. *Toxic epidermal necrolysis*: In which typically sheet like erosions involve more than 30% of the body surface with widespread purpuric macules or flat atypical target lesions, and in which there is severe involvement of mucous membrane (Figs 9.10A and B).
8. *Drug hypersensitivity syndrome (DHS)*: In which rash is often discrete and associated with non-specific multisystem involvement—fever, nausea, vomiting, abdominal pain, diarrhea. Changes in CBC, liver enzymes, LDH, creatinine,

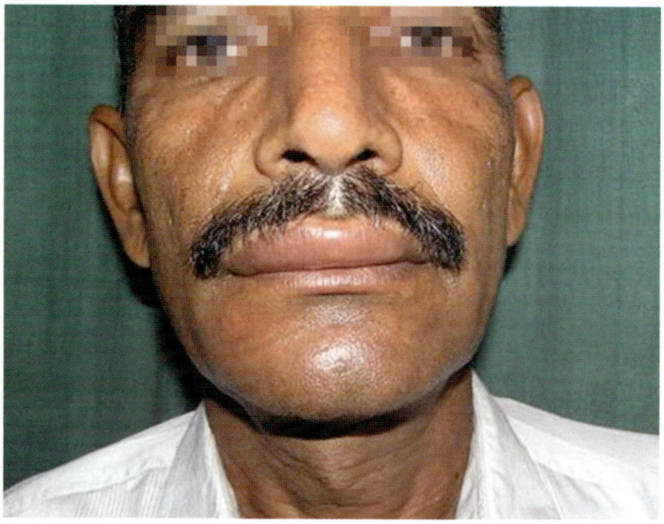

Fig. 9.3: Angioedema

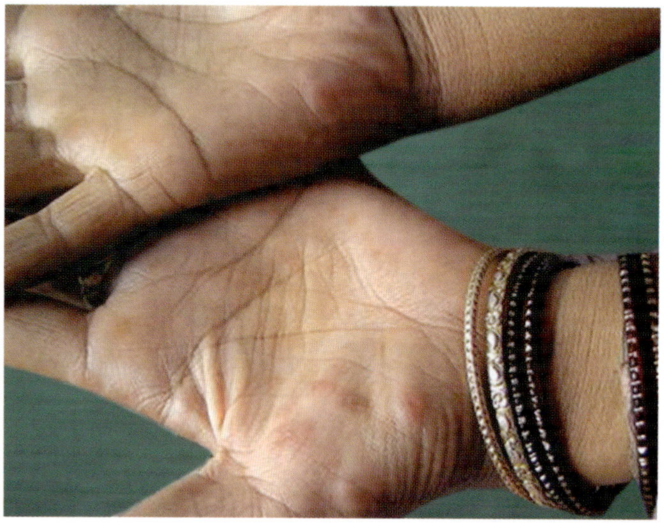

Fig. 9.5: Erythema multiforme over palms

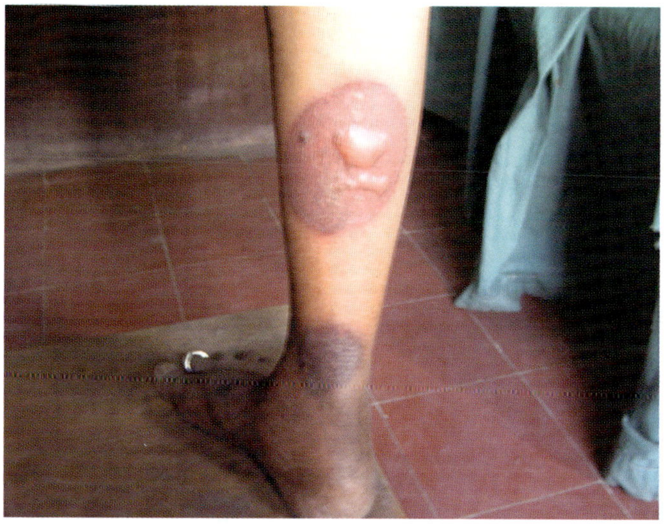

Fig. 9.4: Bullous fixed drug eruption

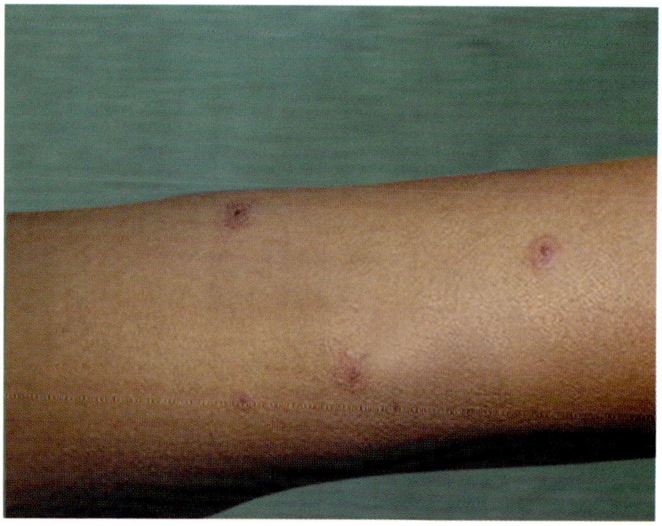

Fig. 9.6: Erythema multiforme over forearm

Abacavir is associated with a potentially fatal DHS in up to 8% of patient. It is associated with particular HLA halotype (HLA B*5701, HLA DR7 and HLA DQ3) efavirenz, delaviridine and amprenavir are also associated with DHS.

9. *Lipodystrophy syndrome*: Protease inhibitors and NRTIs like stavudine may cause it (Figs 9.11A and B).

There is a pattern of central fat accumulation on abdomen, breasts, posterior neck or peripheral fat wasting of face, buttocks and limbs or both.

It is accompanied by hyperlipidemia, lactic acidosis and insulin resistance.

Discontinuation or replacement of PI therapy does not result in reversal of these changes in most patient.

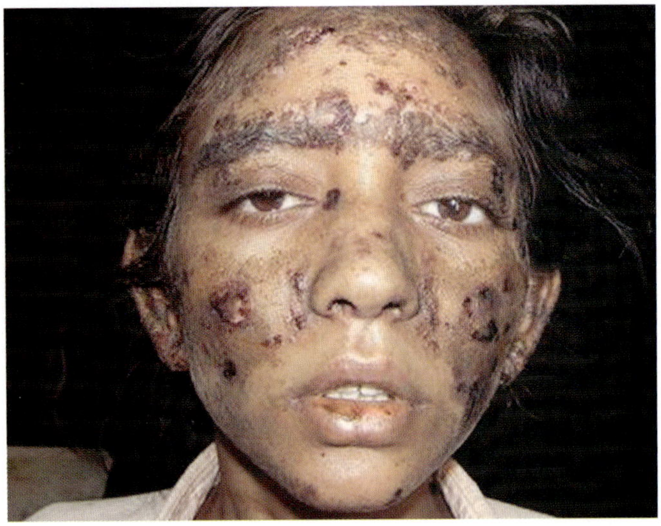

Fig. 9.7: Steven Johnson (SJ) syndrome

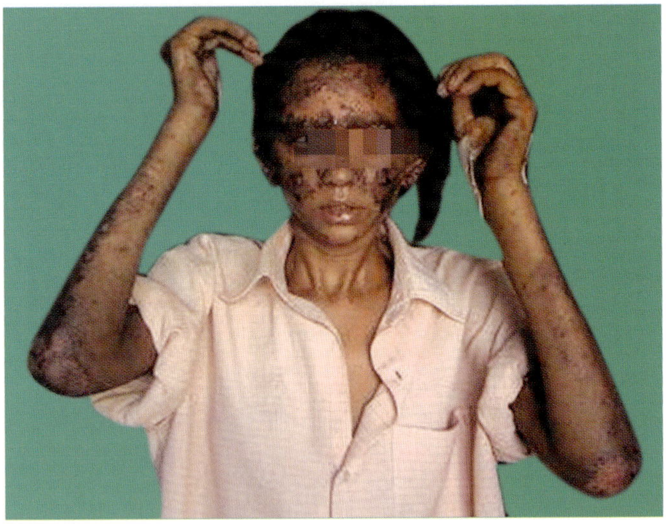

Fig. 9.8 SJ syndrome (Sulfa)

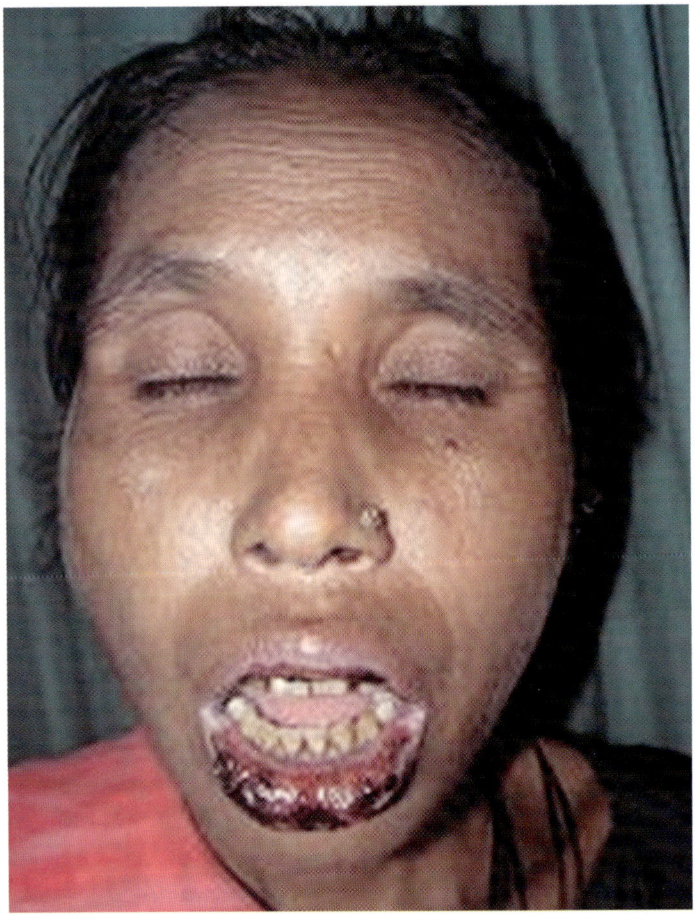

Fig. 9.9: SJ syndrome (NSAID induced)

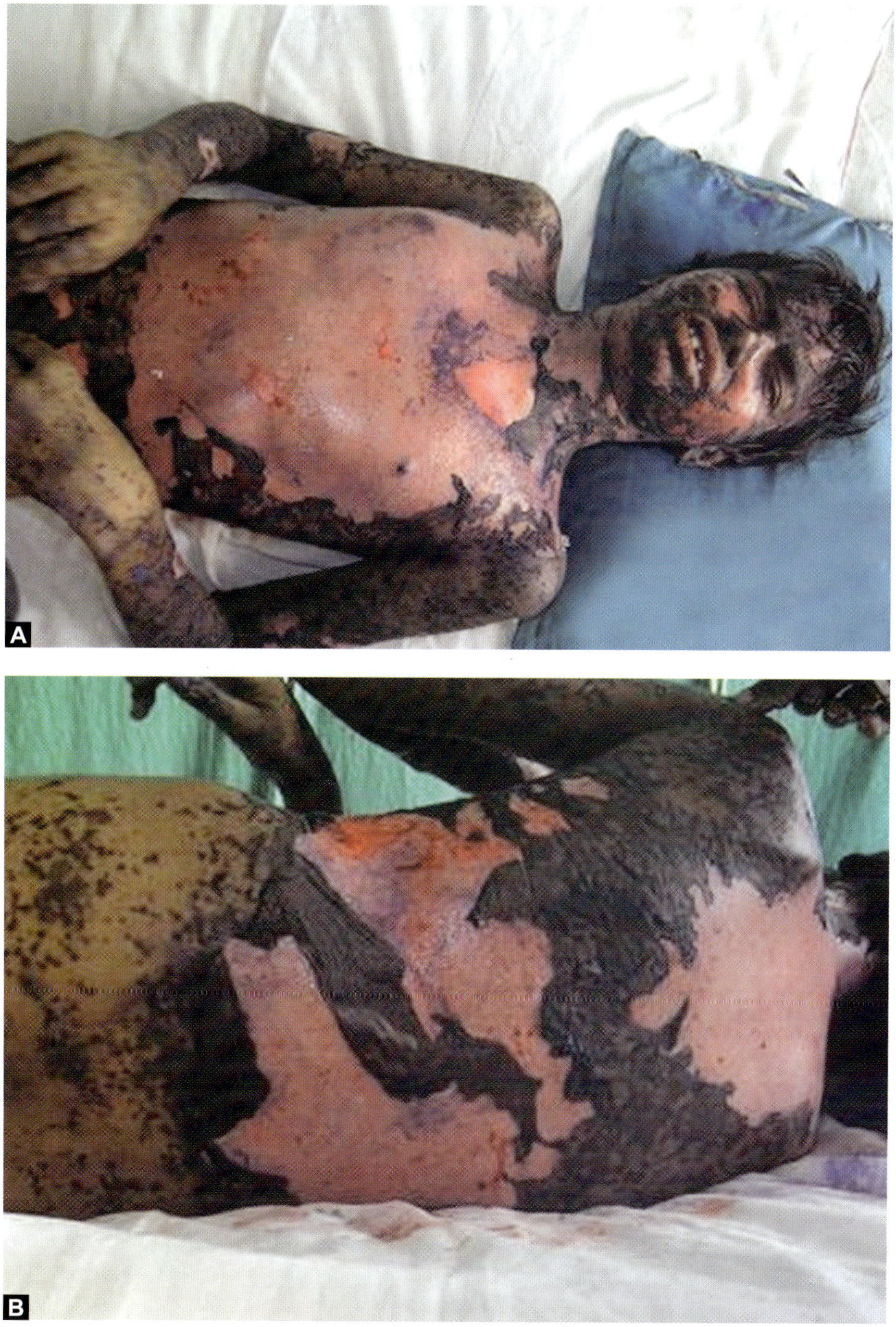

Figs 9.10A and B: Toxic epidermal necrolysis (TEN) (Nevirapine induced)

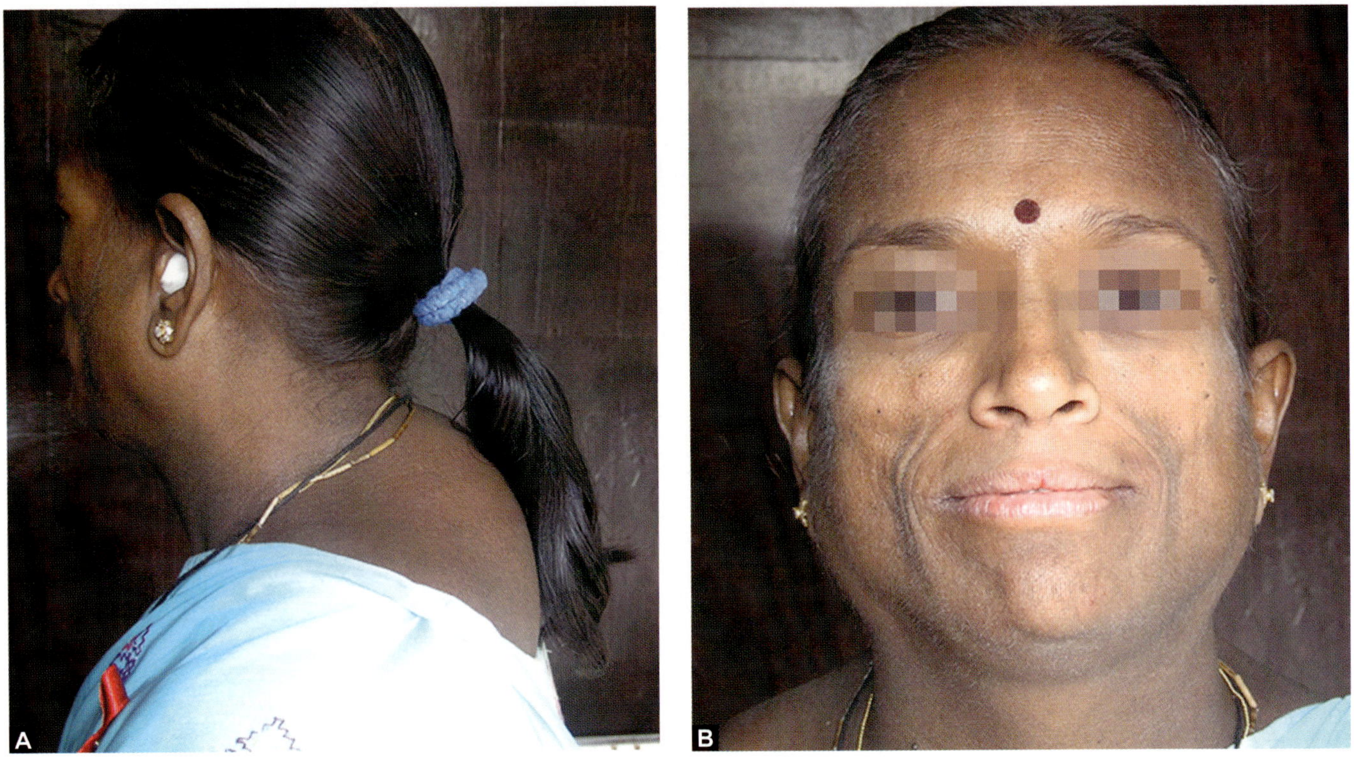

Figs 9.11A and B: Lipodystrophy. (A) Buffalo hump due to indinavir; (B) Lipoatrophy

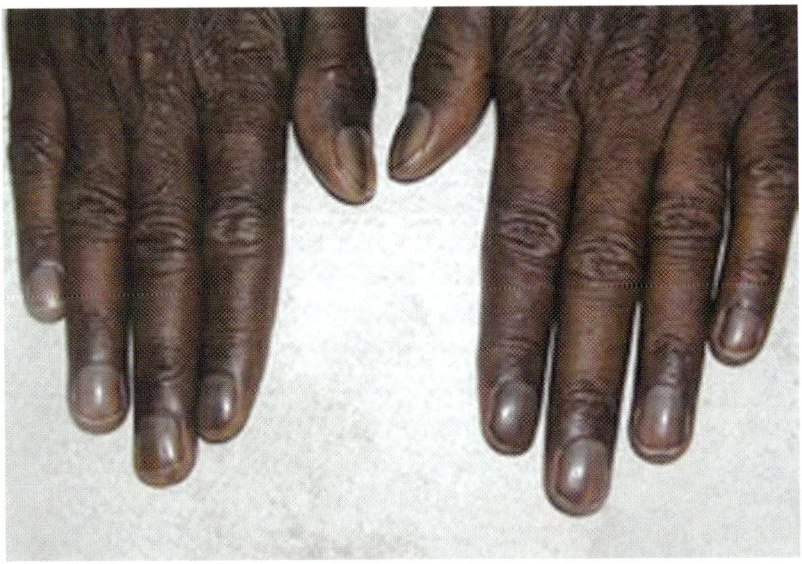

Fig. 9.12: Mucosal pigmentation

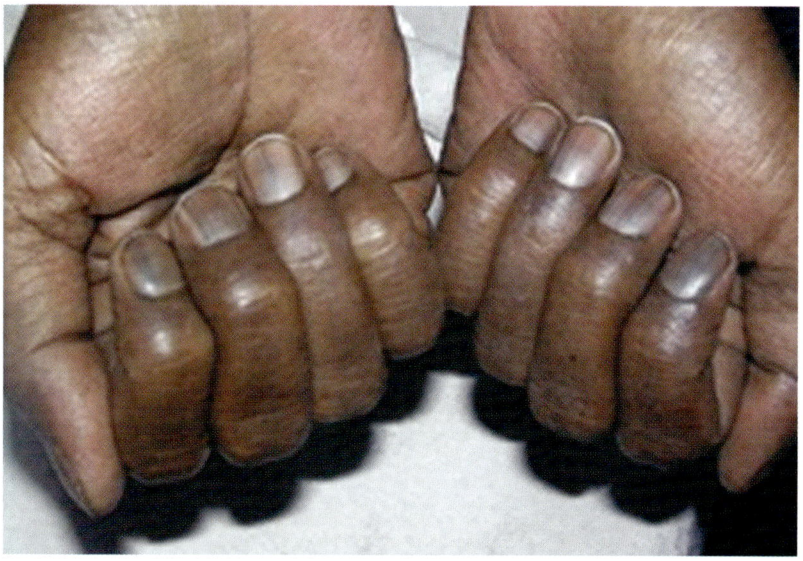

Fig. 9.13: Nail pigmentation

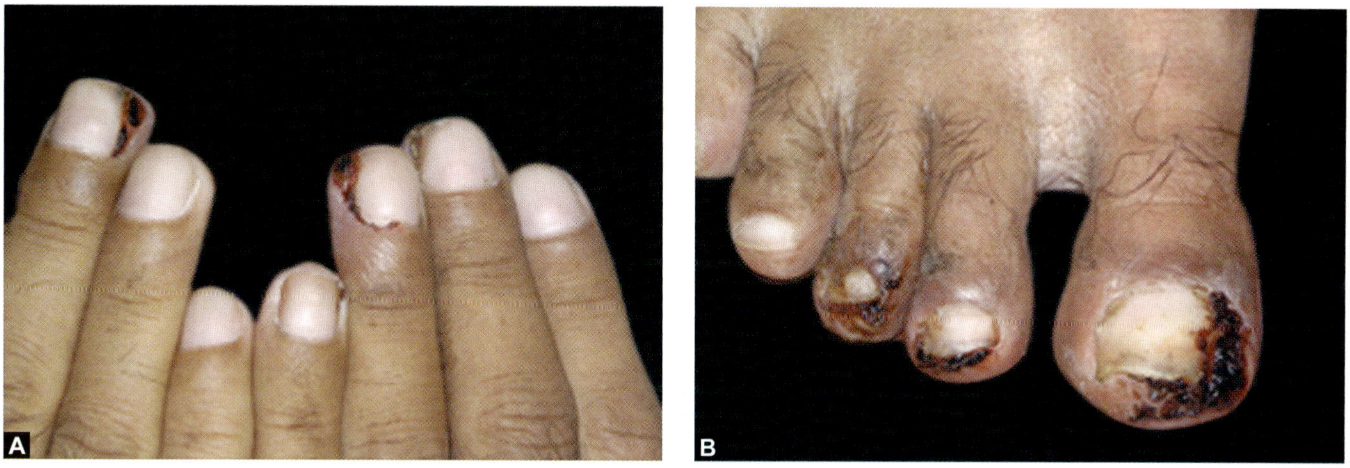

Figs 9.14A and B: Pyogenic granuloma in patient on indinavir

10. *Dress*: Drug rash eosinophillia and systemic symptoms.
11. *Nail pigmentation*: Zidovudine commonly causes longitudinal brown streak of hyperpigmentation of nail plate (Fig. 9.13).
12. *Pyogenic granuloma*: It is caused by indinavir (Figs 9.14A and B).

Various other side effects that have been seen and reported with use of antiretroviral drugs are:
- Cheilitis
- Dryness
- Leukocytoclastic vasculitis
- Mucosal pigmentation (Fig. 9.12)
- Acne.

Index

Page numbers followed by *f* refer to figure